# Warfare the Weight!

How to Achieve Supernatural Weight Loss Through Prayer!

Peggy Lee

## DEDICATION

Dedicated to my Lord and Savior Jesus Christ.
Thank you Lord, for saving my soul and setting me free from
my weight issues.

# CONTENTS

# ACKNOWLEDGMENTS

Thank you Melissa.

You never let me give up on believing God for the opportunity
to share this revelation with the Body of Christ.

# INTRODUCTION

Before we start, I want to make a bit of a disclaimer. Truthfully, this teaching is geared towards instructing intercessors, prayer warriors, ministers and mature Believers in Christ that have a working knowledge of the Word of God.

Why so "exclusive"? Because the spiritual nature of this teaching is pretty intense and some of these truths might be misunderstood by those who are not familiar with the concept of spiritual warfare. Also I'll be sharing this information using Biblical terms and principles that I am going to assume you, the reader, are already familiar with. Understand please that there's simply not time to go over elementary principles here, we've got weight to lose and health to gain, so hopefully you'll be able to jump right in!

You see if we as leaders in the Body of Christ can grasp these truths, we can then turn around and share this in a gentle and loving way with new or immature Believers. Those who may need this information but may not be able to take it all in without being offended or confused or worse yet, scared, thinking the devil is "possessing" them or something silly like that. But since you are spiritual leaders, I can be confident that you will be able to understand the bigger picture here of how the enemy works and then, share what you learn today with others. . . on whatever spiritual level they may be on at the time. Amen?

Ok then. . .

Now that we have established that this teaching is for mature Believers and leaders in the Body. . . Believers who are not easily offended (hopefully) I want to begin by assuring you that there is no condemnation in this message!

You see, not too many years ago, I weighed almost 100 pounds more than I do now. I was a Youth Pastor, involved in prayer ministry and was teaching two Bible studies a week. Oh, I was "spiritual" . . . but I was trapped in a body I hated.

So I need you to know, that I'm not saying anyone with a weight issue, is not spiritual enough!

I would and will never put any type of condemnation on anyone in any way for being overweight. Because I've been there!

My purpose in all this, is simply to share what I have learned in my weight loss journey with others, because I hope it will bless you and, because I know it works!

And I'm not saying that in pride, I'm saying that in complete confidence in the Lord and His Power and the Principles within the Word of God. And, because I know firsthand that this power can be applied to our weight loss efforts to bring about supernatural success!

You see, I have been teaching on this subject matter for many years and the truths I'm about to share are the truths I tapped into to lose that 100 pounds. And while I have taught this in different formats, I feel the Lord has fined tuned this information into the format that I'm about to share with you here, for this specific spiritual season in time. Why?

Because the Holy Spirit prompted me to re-teach this in this particular way, after we began dealing with the Corona virus.

And I know that most of you know this truth but let me share an excerpt from an article off of the WEBMD website, dated July 14th, 2020. It reads like this:

> It has become clearer that people who are obese are one of the groups at highest risk from the disease, regardless of their age. The CDC recently refined its risk categories for COVID-19, stating that obesity was as big a risk for COVID as having a suppressed immune system or chronic lung or kidney disease.

Ok, now remember, that we are mature Believers and spiritual leaders, and we know better than to get offended, right?

Because I'm about to address "the elephant in the room" that to my knowledge, no one wants to talk about.

Church. . . we have a problem.

And that problem is, that the majority of Believers are overweight!

The last statistic I read said that 65% of those who call themselves "born again Believers" are either near, or in, the weight BMI (Body Mass Index) category of what is considered "obese"!

65% of us!

And what makes it so bad, is, that WE ARE THE ONES WHO HAVE THE POWER OF GOD! We have the same power that raised Jesus from the dead! We have the mighty rushing wind power of the Holy Spirit!

However, for the most part, this seems to be a problem we just can't overcome!

And I "go there" because I believe the Lord is, in a sense, "sounding an alarm" for us in this area!

But before you get defensive, let me just say, that what He has told me, is that He is NOT expecting us to all to be "beauty queens and body builders"!

**HE JUST WANTS US TO TRY!** To try to put out some effort in this area and to address this issue in a serious manner.

You see I believe that the virus has made it clear that we need to put our health right at the **TOP** of our list of "natural" priorities!

Now of course, our relationship with the Lord must always come first – sure! But as Christians, I believe the Lord is really calling us to come up higher in a lot of ways and to put more focus on this subject and how it affects our lives. I mean think about it...

Without your health, your physical body is essentially out of commission! And...

- Without your physical body you can't fulfill your ministry!
- Without your physical body you can't walk out your destiny!
- Without your physical body you can't live to see your life blessed and get married, have kids and grandkids and participate in those type things that Lord wants you to enjoy!

Friends, according to the CDC, obesity is the number one contributor to Heart disease and Diabetes. And, it's the secondary contributor to many other serious health issues!

So I'm sorry to be the one to have to bring this to your attention, but obesity is pre-maturely taking out the Body of Christ one, by one, by one.

Heart attack, Diabetes, Corona Virus, . . . gone, gone, gone!

Church, as Christians it's time we faced this issue and begin to take a stand against it! A stand both in the natural realm *and* in the Spirit realm, amen?

Let me remind you that the Bible says your body is "the temple of the Holy Spirit" (1 Corinthians 6:19). Well, that makes it a sacred thing, wouldn't you say?

So my question to you is this. Why, why, why, do we abuse our bodies like we do?

Why do we do things and eat things we know we shouldn't do and eat. . . and why do *not* do things and *not* eat the type of things that we know we should?

Let me answer that question for you in a way you may have never thought of before.

Friend, I want to remind you that we are in an all-out war down here with demonic entities in the invisible spirit realm that hate us!

Look with me at this verse:

## John 10:10 New International Version

The thief comes only to steal and kill and destroy; I have come that they may have life and have it to the full.

Church, we KNOW this verse! But let's put it into this context.

Think. What is the devil's "job"? To steal, kill and destroy, correct?

And, what is a major problem within the Body of Christ right now? Being overweight, correct?

Well, what does being overweight do to our health?

It STEALS, KILLS AND DESTROYS IT, right?

So whose fingerprints are all over this situation? The enemy's! That's who!

Now let's think this through some more...

Why do we pray against the devil for everything under the sun, but completely ignore his influence when it comes to *this* area of our life?

I have heard mighty men and women of God say one minute, "Nothing is impossible with God!" and then turn around a few minutes later and say, "I just *can't* lose this extra weight"!

Church, what has happened to us in this area? It's like we've had these huge blinders on!

We look down our holy noses at the drug addicts and the prostitutes, but yet *we* have "fellowships" for every event under the sun and laugh about our addiction to eating like it's no big deal. When the truth is, that we are eating ourselves into an early grave!

So back to the devil.

I have a question for you.

If a drug addict came to you as a spiritual leader and said, "I want to get delivered, I want to get set free, I want to get myself cleaned up, I don't want to live this way anymore..."

If they said that to you, what would you do?

You'd pray right? And you'd probably come against that spirit of addiction and you'd bind it and break its power and then, you'd probably pray forth an anointing of freedom and blessing onto their life, correct?

Well, church. . . same devil, different problem.

It's time that we as Believers see this issue for the spiritual situation that it is, and begin to PRAY INTO OURSELVES, strategically. . . until all the extra weight is gone and we are "set free", cleaned up and have achieved peace in this area of our life!

And that's the purpose of this teaching because that's exactly what I did. I dug into the Word of God, crafted a strategic prayer and began to pray it every day, until all the extra weight came off.

And I want you to know that if you will just get serious about this and begin to implement the things I'm about to share with you, the extra weight that you are carrying will come off of you too!

In fact, allow me to decree over you now, that from this time forward, the Lord is going to empower you, and enable you to become an "overcomer" in this area of your life!

Look with me at these verses.

### Revelation 2:7 (New King James)
To him who overcomes I will give to eat from the tree of life. . .

### Revelation 2:17 (New King James)
To him who overcomes I will give some of the hidden manna . . .

### Revelation 2:26 (New King James)
And he who overcomes. . . I will give power over the nations. . .

### Revelation 3:5 (New King James)
He who overcomes, shall be clothed in white garments. . .

As Believers, we are called to overcome anything and everything that is coming against us in life! So why do we lay down in defeat when it comes to the issue of being overweight?

**I'M HERE TO TELL YOU TO RISE UP!**

It's time to put on that Rocky Theme music, get your fighting clothes on, and come against this situation like the overcomer you are!

I need you to realize today that it is **NOT** God's perfect will for you to be trapped in an overweight body that makes you miserable!

Is it His "permissive" will? Sure! He'll **LET** you eat and eat and eat and lay on the couch all day, until you weigh **500** pounds. He's not going to slap the food out of your hand, is He?

However, do you think a mighty man or woman of God weighing 500 pounds is God's **PERFECT** will for that person?

No! Why?

Because the extra weight on that body is ultimately bondage! It's mental, emotional and actual physical bondage that we are carrying around with us, day in and day out. And it's not God's perfect will for His people to be in **ANY** type of Bondage, is it?

Friends, God's perfect will for you is to be in a lean, strong, healthy body for your frame size. And that will be different for each of us.

You see, when it comes down to it, it's not about a number on the scale. It's about being physically well able to function in a body that you feel good about.

A body that doesn't cause you grief.

That's what God wants for you! And that's what He can enable you to have *if* you just start to apply His Power and His Principles to this area of your life!

Church, we have got more work to do right now for the Kingdom of God than we have ever had before! And I believe with all my heart that God is raising up a mighty army to do that work.

And what's the first thing that a soldier goes through when they enlist in the Army? Boot camp, right?

And boot camp consists of a time of seriously focused, physical training. It's a time when that out of shape young man or lady gets themself in the kind of physical condition that they never dreamed they could achieve!

And it's tough…but when it's over, they feel STRONG AND EMPOWERED! Because they are physically ready to go to war!

Well friend, I believe that's what we're stepping into right now!

God's Army needs to address the issue of its weight problem that we've been sweeping under the rug. And we need to put ourselves in a self-imposed, "boot camp" so to speak, so that we become lean, mean, fighting machines for the Kingdom of God!

Friends I've been seeking the Lord on this subject for a long time. And the Lord told me years ago, that "one day" . . . He was going to bring about a "Fitness Revival" within the Body of Christ. Well, I honestly believe that time has come!

So I'm telling you today with love and compassion in my heart, that it's time for us to get serious about our weight issues and attack this problem AT THE ROOT!

And that's what you're going to do with this strategy!

I'm going to give you a prayer outline to pray each day and then I'm going to explain the prayer and show you how to "walk it out" by applying it to your eating and exercise habits.

It's really amazingly easy. And because I know that it worked for me, I am confident in saying that the power that the prayer releases will also work for you!

You see, I want you to realize today that Father God is ready, willing and able to help you in this area! And, He is a God that works both supernaturally *and* suddenly, right?

Well if you're in agreement with that, let me add one more thing as I finish up this chapter and it's this.

The Lord has told me that even as you read all of this, before you even begin to take action on it, but as you go over it in your mind and think through these principles being applied to your weight issues, that **HIS POWER** for weight loss is going to be released!

Yes, the anointing for weight loss will be released through the revelation as you read it and take it into your spirit! So get ready to experience that wonderful result in your life!

Now, with all that said, my exhortation to you today is this. If you will just decide right now that losing weight and getting yourself in better physical condition is something that you need to get serious about. . . then I'm here to tell you, that the Lord is going to meet your decision with His Presence and flood your actions with **HIS SUPERNATURAL POWER!**

And He will, from this time on, work with you to transform your body into a body you feel good about -- so that you are physically well able to fulfill your particular ministry or calling from the Lord!

Does that sound like something you can get on board with? Great! Then let's begin!

# THE ENEMY'S PART

Friend, if being overweight is a negative thing, and if it "steals, kills and destroys" our health and the quality of our life, then why have we not realized that there are demonic forces behind it?

This is where we have missed it!

This is why we haven't been able to lose weight, feel great and stay healthy! Because we haven't been approaching this issue in the right way!

You see for the most part, we've been coming against the effects... but not the cause!

Look with me at these verses. Luke 13:10-13 first out of the New King James version and then, out of the Passion Translation.

### Luke 13:10-13 New King James Version

Now He was teaching in one of the synagogues on the Sabbath. <sup>11</sup>And behold, there was a woman who had a spirit of infirmity eighteen years and was bent over and could in no way raise herself up. [12] But when Jesus saw her, He called her to Him and said to her, "Woman, you are loosed from your infirmity." [13] And He laid His hands on her, and immediately she was made straight, and glorified God.

Now, let's look at that out of the Passion Translation:

### Luke 13:10-13 The Passion Translation

[10] One Sabbath day, while Jesus was teaching in the synagogue, [11] he encountered a seriously handicapped woman. She was crippled and had been doubled over for eighteen years. Her condition was caused by a demonic spirit of bondage that had left her unable to stand up straight.

When Jesus saw her condition, he called her over and gently laid his hands on her. Then he said, "Dear woman, you are free. I release you forever from this crippling spirit." Instantly she stood straight and tall and overflowed with glorious praise to God!

Ok, Believers let's think.

We see here that this woman's "condition" was caused by a demonic spirit. . . and when Jesus simply acknowledged it, confronted it and spoke against it, it left and immediately her condition changed!

Well, THIS is what you are about to do concerning your "condition" of being overweight!

But first, let's review what we know about demonic spirits.

Now I'm not an expert but to my knowledge, demons are spiritual entities that have, for lack of a better way to put it, "personalities".

You see demonic spirits embody particular "traits" or characteristics and they basically work 24 hours a day trying to influence people to manifest that trait.

For instance, what we would call a "spirit of anger", tries to get people to agree with it and react to a particular situation with anger. And if he fools that person into expressing anger, then that particular spirit is satisfied, because it's accomplished it's goal.

So understand please, that demonic spirits have assignments. It's just a fact in the Spirit realm. And to put that in this context, let me suggest to you this.

What if. . . there is a whole "group" of spirits that work, 24/7 to make and keep us overweight?

What if they *know*. . . how easily we can be tempted to overeat and to not be physically active and they simply play right into our weaknesses, day in and day out, *knowing* that an overweight, out of shape, Christian loses his or her "edge'.

And what does that mean?

It means we're just not as "sharp" as we could be! The extra weight slows us down, makes us uncomfortable, works negatively on our self-confidence and, often opens spiritual doors for other demonic spirits of sickness and disease to enter into our life!

Now I realize that's some heavy stuff there but hang with me for a bit. You see, I believe with all my heart that there is, this group of demonic entities working against us. And because of that, I want you to know today that your weight problem is NOT all your fault!

What if I told you that we have, unknowingly, been influenced by forces in the invisible spirit realm that work diligently against us. They work to influence us to overeat, to eat the wrong type of foods, and make and keep us so tired that we just don't want to exercise. And while that sounds a bit alarming, what we have to realize is this.

IF... there are demonic forces causing a situation to manifest in a negative, harmful way then as Believers, we can and are supposed to, TAKE THOSE SPIRITS OUT!

And that's what we are going to do in the first part of our daily prayer. (I will go over the various sections of the prayer within the text of this book, but I'll give you several "tear out" copies of the entire prayer at the end of the book.)

So anyway. . . what are these spirits you might ask?

Well, I have studied this subject for a lot of years so I'm going to show you the ones that, to the best of my knowledge, affect every aspect of our weight loss efforts. And you can add or subtract to this list if you want. But I promise you, IF you will begin to take authority over these spirits and bind and break their power, YOU WILL SEE RESULTS!

Remember, Luke 10:19 tells us that Jesus has given us authority over every work of the enemy, right? Well, that's what we are about to tap into here!

And while we don't know the exact methodology of *how* they influence us, I feel, we don't really have to! If we will just bind them and command them to leave us, they will go! Amen?

So let's take a look.

The first one is the Spirit of Heaviness. But before we go over this, let me tell you just how this revelation came about.

You see, I was crying one day.... years ago.... and I was feeling fat and miserable and depressed and gross... not able to fit into any of my clothes and basically just wanting to jump off a bridge because I was so bloated and uncomfortable. And I'm praying as I'm crying and I said to the Lord, in tears, "Lord WHYYYY can't I lose weight?"

And after I asked that I heard the Lord's voice, loud and clear, deep down within my spirit, and He said to me this;

"THE SPIRIT OF HEAVINESS"!

Let me show it to you in the Word.

### Isaiah 61:3 (New King James)

To console those who mourn in Zion,

To give them beauty for ashes,

The oil of joy for mourning,

The garment of praise for the spirit of heaviness. . .

Ok, hold onto to that verse in your mind as I finish my story.

When the Lord spoke this to me, truthfully, I was shocked.

You see, I had been a Bible teacher for a lot of years at this point. I loved the Book of Isaiah and had taught from it many times. So, just like everyone else, I had always interpreted the "heaviness" in chapter 61 to mean a type of depression. An "emotional" heaviness *only*. But because the Lord had spoken it to my spirit, I looked it up again. And what I found out, was that the Hebrew word for heaviness means, "to be made darkened, dim, weakened **OR TO BE MADE HEAVY!**

That's the definition of the Hebrew word!

And to take it a step further, the Greek definition from the Vine's Expository Dictionary means, "to be troubled, greatly distressed of mind, to be full of heaviness, or **TO BE HEAVY**"!

So can you see it friend?  It's been "a thing" all along!

Yes, it is attributed in the Word there in Isaiah to an emotional heaviness, but the definition that describes the word referring to the spirit, includes "**TO BE HEAVY**"!

So grab hold of this, because you have to know what it is that you are going to be fighting against!

Church, the spirit of "heaviness" is the spirit that makes something heavy in a negative way! We see it in the Word, working mentally and emotionally so why would we think it could not affect us **PHYSICALLY** too?

Demonic spirits have distinct personalities, assignments and power, right?  So wouldn't it stand to reason that if a spirit of heaviness can "weigh us down" emotionally, that it could "weigh us down" physically as well?

I mean think about how these two areas are related.  I know, beyond a shadow of doubt that the most depressed I've ever been, was because I was so overweight or "heavy".  The

"physical heaviness" brought on the "emotional heaviness".
Can anyone relate to that?

Ok then, look at this -- it can work in reverse too!

When we get down, discouraged and depressed about
something... what's the first thing we usually do? EAT, right?

You break up with your boyfriend, you grab a gallon of ice
cream and a spoon! You get laid off at your job, you come home
and grab a bag of chips and some dip! We go to our "comfort"
foods to make us "feel better" don't we? And that's completely
understandable. Yes, we need that serotonin boost at times but
in reality, by doing this, we are giving this spirit an even tighter
hold upon our lives!

Look, I'm sure any psychologist would tell us that many, many
people are overweight because they use food as a means of
solace and / or protection from emotional trauma and
wounding. So can you see the connection? And can you see
how that spirit of Heaviness could be able to affect both the
emotional *and* physical areas of our lives?

Ok then, back to my point. When I asked the Lord why I
couldn't lose weight, He said to me "the spirit of Heaviness".
And I want you to know today, that *this* is the spirit that is
keeping you overweight too!

You are too "HEAVY" . . . because a SPIRIT OF

"HEAVINESS" has been influencing your mind, your emotions *and* your physical body!

But…just like with ANY demonic spirit, you have the power and authority through Christ to make it leave! Praise God!

Friend, I want you to take a minute here to grasp the enormity of this truth! Because once you start to bind and break the power of this spirit and command it to leave you, IT MUST GO!

And I'm telling you, within a few days you'll start to feel the change in your body! And then as you persevere in prayer, you'll see a whole new body image begin to come forth!

Look with me now at this picture:

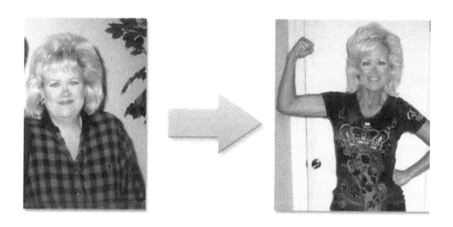

The Peggy on the left unknowingly had the spirit of Heaviness working effectively in her life. But the Peggy on the right, started praying against it, and has never stopped!

(And no I was not pregnant in that first picture … I just looked like it! Ugh!)

So anyway... the spirit of Heaviness is the first and I feel, the most important spirit you will be prompted to take authority over daily.

And I say the "most important" because my theory about it is this.

Since *that's* the one the Lord spoke to me about. . . in my mind, I just feel that maybe it's the main one and that's why the Lord told me about it when I cried out to Him like I did.

But look, I'm not trying to make up some new, weird "doctrine" here. And I promise you I am not "obsessed" with the devil, because I know through Christ, he is a defeated foe.

All I know is, that when I asked the Lord, with tears flowing down my face, "why" I couldn't lose weight, that is what I heard Him say to me. So to me, that's reason enough to take authority over it every day in Jesus' name! Amen?

Ok, the next spirit I want to bring your attention to this. The spirit of "overeating".

Now I call this "overeating" because to me, it's a term we can easily relate to. However, I get this term, and the revelation of it being a spirit we need to deal with for weight loss, from this verse:

### Proverbs 23:1-3 New International Version

When you sit to dine with a ruler,

note well what is before you,

and put a knife to your throat

if you are given to GLUTTONY.

That version is kind of harsh, huh? But the truth is, that the Bible does indeed talk about "gluttony" and look at how it describes it here. It says "IF. . . you are "given to gluttony" . . . which says to me, that some people are given to it, but we don't have to be!

Now before we go on, let me share my "Little Debbie" story. Because again, I want to assure you there is no condemnation in this teaching coming from me, at all!

You see, I believe now, that I am a recovered "glutton". Which means according to that verse that we just read, I should have put a knife to my throat. . . but I didn't. Instead I just cried out to God and began to dig into the Word!

Remember at the time that picture on the left (from the previous page) was taken, like I said before, I loved the Lord, I was faithful in church and I was teaching the Word of God.

But for my breakfast... every day. . . for *years*...I would have, do you know those Little Debbie swiss cake rolls? You know how there are two of those delicious little preservative filled critters in each wonderful pack?

Well, I would have EVERY. SINGLE. DAY. . .
as soon as I woke up....
Not one... two pack of little Debbie's...
Not two, two packs of little Debbie's...
But three two packs of Little Debbie's, making a grand total of 6 Little Debbie swiss cake rolls EVERY SINGLE MORNING for my breakfast! Ugh!

Yes, I had issues friends! And with that much sugar how to you think I felt about 3 o'clock? Not good, I promise you!

So again, I am not judging anyone! I'm just here to share with you what I found out! So, back to that issue of gluttony.

We see it in the Word, but because "gluttony" is not a term we like to use much, I'm just going to call it a spirit of "overeating". Because the truth is, that as Christians, we truly need to acknowledge that it's something very, very real!

And why is that so?

Well…. because in this day of unlimited availability of fast food, snack foods and microwave quick fix food, the truth is, that eating way beyond the amount of food we actually *need* is truly a problem!

In fact, if we step back and look at the big picture, we can see how eating related sin may just be the number one temptation overall that Believers deal with. Let's think about this. . .

Church, do you realize that the very first sin involved eating? When Satan tempted Eve in the garden, he tempted her to eat something she should not have eaten, correct?

Well don't you know his methods never really change?

I mean we know the Lord has given us food to nourish our bodies and to enjoy with our taste buds, but isn't it just like the enemy to take something God made for good and exploit it to excess so that it becomes something bad?

Bad for us health-wise, contributing to Heart disease, Diabetes and such, and also bad for us emotionally and mentally, because the extra weight on our bodies, caused mostly from overeating, contributes to the trap of the almost universal problem called, "low self- esteem"!

So my theory, as I was developing this prayer strategy was this:

*IF* there are demonic spirits working their best to influence us to overeat, would it not be worth taking a minute or so to pray and bind them, just in case? So that if they are "real" they wouldn't be able to operate in your life that day?

Well that's what I started to do, and that's what I suggest you do also. Because I promise you, they ARE real. And as you begin to break their power, you will be amazed at the difference in your eating habits and how the prayer brings supernatural results! Yay Jesus!

Ok, let's go on.

The next spirit you will bind each day is this: The spirit of "tiredness".

Now we know that people got tired even back in Bible times, and I get that. It's just a natural side effect of living life in a human body, for sure! So, while I've never read in the Word where it mentions a "spirit of tiredness" per se, my thought is, why are we all always so tired? Could there possibly be some undesirable spiritual forces ADDING TO that symptom? I think that could be so. Look with me at this verse.

<u>Proverbs 19:15 English Standard Version</u>
Slothfulness casts into a deep sleep. . .

Now this word slothfulness in the Hebrew means inactive,

lethargic, drowsy and of little energy. So, what I'm calling a "spirit of tiredness" in this prayer, may actually be the spirit behind the slothfulness that we see here in the Word. Because these days you can ask pretty much anyone, at any time of day, if they're "tired" (of little energy) and 9 times out of 10 they will say, "yes"!

So IF there are demonic forces at play, and I believe there are…then why not pray against that spirit's attribute affecting your body? Well, that's just what we'll do, every day, through our daily prayer! Now again, you'll see exactly how we pray this when we go over the entire prayer, but for now, let's go on.

The next "spirit of" you will take authority over, will be what I call, the spirit of "excess hunger and food cravings".

You see while the spirit of gluttony makes us eat too much, as in too large of portions, I believe there are also spirits similar to the gluttony spirit who work in a little bit different way. So we will be addressing here the spirits that tempt us to stress eat, emotionally eat, eat out of boredom and eat as the result of a "craving". Because I am convinced there are spirits that prompt us, in our minds, to do these things that we have for years just mindlessly obeyed!

And why have we done that? Because we just *assumed* it was

our own thoughts making us want to eat in this way, correct?

But what if it's not?

Church, we have to be knowledgeable about how the demonic realm works, so that we can stay ahead of it. And the truth is that there are spirits assigned to you, your family and your bloodline, who not only study you, but are patient enough to wait until the perfect time to "hook ya" with their deception and lies.

So let's bring this generality into this specific aspect of our eating habits. You know, the eating habits that continually sabotage your weight loss efforts in whatever way they can?

Friend what if, there are spirits who know you well enough to know that IF you are stressed, IF you are emotionally upset, or IF you are bored, you will follow their lead right into the kitchen and eat until you "feel better"?

This is the kind of "hunger" will be dealing with here. That "extra" in between meal eating, that you don't need and truthfully don't really even want!

And I hate to step on your toes here, but let's take a minute to more closely examine that "extra" eating.

What motivation could the enemy be using to get us to partake of this type of eating?  Let me suggest, two hidden psychological triggers that possibly could be in the enemy's arsenal belt.

The first is what I call "self- indulgence".  It's closely linked with pride in that, it is the emotional hook that causes one to think, "I deserve this!".

Had a bad day?  Stop at the bakery and pick up some cupcakes. Why?  "I deserve this, because I had a bad day!".

You see the underlying truth in this mindset is that "I deserve to gratify my flesh (which is your sin nature) because of this stressful situation that I had to deal with!"  "It was hard, and I didn't like it", so I'm going to give my flesh exactly what fattening foods it wants, because. . . (and then we insert any number of excuses in this spot!)".

Friend, can you see what the enemy has done in this case? He attacks you and gives you something difficult to go through and then he feeds the thought in your mind that you "deserve" to do something that will put your body in more bondage "just because".

Now sure, a bit of self-indulgence is of course ok on some

special occasions, but IF… you fall for this trap time and time again, *watch out for it and start to be smart!*

Now the second psychological trigger I believe the enemy uses to bait us is just the opposite. It's self-sabotage or self-hate.

This can come from any number of situations, but it's the mindset that says, "I don't care if this is not good for me, I'm having it anyway because… (and again, we insert our excuses here)".

And with this one, the result is the same. It's you overeating food that you *know* you shouldn't be eating. But the motivation behind this one is self-sabotage because it stems from "not caring" about yourself and your health at that moment in time. And this, like the "I deserve this" mindset, results in you unknowingly working *with* the suggestions of the enemy, to bring the bondage of extra weight and all of its negative ramifications upon yourself.

Think this through. Does any of this apply to you?

Do you sometimes eat out of self-indulgence which says, "I deserve this!", or do you sometimes eat out of self-hatred, which says, "I don't care!"?

Hosea 4:6 says, "My people are destroyed for lack of knowledge". Could this be knowledge that you need to pray through to stop being "destroyed" in this way?

Food for thought! (Sorry, bad pun! ☺)

Now cravings are another thing that run similar to this line of thinking. And I realize that some food cravings are legitimately physiologically based, sure! Our hormones and brain chemicals do some weird things sometimes, as you know if you have ever been pregnant. So that's not what we will address here.

We will address those cravings that we think are ok but are not. Those cravings that might be caused by our playing right into the enemy's hands once again. Let me give you an example.

I had a lady tell me once that she HAD to have ice cream every night before bed because she "craved" it. . . and if she didn't eat the ice cream, the craving was so strong that she just couldn't sleep. Now there may be some kind of nutritional deficiency in play here, but in general, does it sound like a "God thing" to you? Or could that be some trick of the enemy convincing this lady that her "craving" was of her own doing and that if she didn't "obey" it, she wouldn't sleep?

I'm telling you prayer warriors, yes, our "flesh", which is our sin nature, contributes to our overeating and being overweight, of course!  WE yield to our flesh and choose to put the fork up to our mouths.....YES!

But who and what do you think *pulls the strings of our flesh, tempting us* to do these things to ourselves?  The same class of beings who have been tempting mankind since creation, that's who!

Realize today that the enemy works to influence your mind and body so that YOU, PUT YOURSELF in bondage!

He's invisible. . . he can't stick food in your mouth. . . but he can sure play with your mind and your emotions to get YOU to stick the food in your mouth!  And then he laughs at you, because in reality YOU DID IT TO YOURSELF!

However. . . once you start to "warfare the weight" by praying PROACTIVELY in these various ways, the enemy's power will be broken!  So by binding up what I call here, "the spirit of excess hunger and food cravings" every day, I'm telling you, you're going to see the result!

Get ready to coast right through that 4pm chocolate craving, that "have to have" popcorn while watching a movie or that, 'if

I don't eat ice cream I won't sleep" snack at night! Because when you address these things in the SPIRIT REALM, it affects the things in the NATURAL REALM! So you are going to stop just treating the symptoms, but instead, overcome the problem by going straight to the root!

Friend, every time you pray any warfare type prayer, you break the enemy's power off of you! And by targeting *this* particular area of your life in prayer, supernatural weight loss will be the result!

Alrighty! Now with all that said, let's stop right here and review. These are the spirits you will bind daily by following the Warfare the Weight Power Prayer:

- Heaviness
- Overeating
- Tiredness
- Excess hunger and food cravings

If you can think of anymore, feel free to add them. However, I've studied this subject for many years and feel confident this pretty effectively covers the demonic forces and strategies that are working against us to make and keep us overweight! It works for me any way, and I know it will work for you too!

To finish this chapter up, let me show you now, how the first part of the prayer will go.  It reads like this:

*In the name of Jesus, I take authority over every demonic spirit affecting my body, my weight and my health and I render these spirits POWERLESS to operate in my life in Jesus' name!*

*Spirit of Heaviness, Spirit of Overeating, Spirit of Tiredness, and Spirit of Excess hunger and food cravings, I bind you, I break your power, I command you to leave me now in Jesus' name!*

Ok, that's easy enough don't you think? It takes like what? 30 seconds?

Friend, I promise you it's **WELL WORTH** the 30 seconds it takes to use the authority Jesus has given you and stop these intruders from interfering in this area of your life!

I'll close by showing you this quote from Martin Luther King Jr., that I think is so powerful. It says,

"Freedom is never voluntarily given by the oppressor; it must be demanded by the oppressed." - Martin Luther King, Jr.

Church, this is a Spiritual truth!

Those spirits are never going to leave you alone until you **MAKE THEM** leave you! Amen?  And that's just what you'll do by praying this daily prayer! Praise the Lord!

# THE HOLY SPIRIT - YOUR PERSONAL TRAINER

Now that we've gotten all the negative forces bound up and powerless, let's get to fun part!

I want you to realize that as Believers, the supernatural should be our natural! We should be so used to living a life filled with God's power that everything we do should be producing supernatural results! Well, that's the mindset and the power that you're about to tap into.

You see, the power of the Holy Spirit within you is ready, willing and able to operate in your life in any and every way possible. So why not put Him to work full time in the weight loss area of your life?

According to John 14:26, He is the "helper" you know?? So do you not think He wants to help you in this area too?

Friends think about it. Your weight issues pretty much affect every other part of your life! Because again, it's bondage.

Mental, emotional, and physical bondage! And bondage restricts your freedom. But Jesus came to set the captives free, did He not?

And doesn't 2 Corinthians 3:17 reveal to us, that "where the Spirit of the Lord is there is freedom"?

Well here's the trick. When you plug the Spirit of the Lord into this situation, FREEDOM WILL BE THE RESULT!

But just to clarify, let me make a bit of a disclaimer here.

Everyone is not going to be a size 4 skinny-minny or a men's belt size 30. This is not about the people of God striving for what the world calls, "perfection". Oh no, no, no, no!

In fact, this may seem hard to believe, but the truth is, that some of God's children would fall into great pride if they truly reached a number on the scale that they say, they would like to reach. . . because their new body image would ultimately work to be a prideful hindrance in their lives. So please understand that this isn't about looking good in a bikini or looking better than your co-worker that you don't like. No.

This is about you living in a body that you are comfortable in and can get around easily enough to be able to physically fulfill your destiny in Christ.

And, it's about getting to a place of having peace in this area so that this issue is no longer a stronghold in your mind and in your life!

So, if the extra weight on your body is hindering your physical ability and your emotional well-being, then it needs to go! And it will. Because what you will be doing, will be done so that you can be lean, strong and healthy for the Glory of God.

And the great news is, that the Holy Spirit can and will, lead, guide, direct and empower you to lose the extra weight on your body and get healthy! All it takes on your end is to ASK HIM… and THEN be willing to follow His lead.

Ok…

Let me show you now, the middle section of the daily prayer. After you have bound and broke the power of the various spirits that we previously discussed each day, next you will pray something like this:

*Now, Holy Spirit I ask you today to be my Personal Trainer. Lead, guide and direct me in my eating and exercise habits and empower me to lose this extra weight and become supernaturally healthy, in Jesus' name!*

We will discuss in detail the "eating and exercise habits" in another section. But what I want you to know right now is, that the Holy Spirit of God is an absolute genius concerning any and every subject -- even the subject of weight loss!

Because friend, He knows you inside out!

He sees your biological and chemical makeup and knows exactly what and how much you should eat. And, He knows every aspect of your physical body and its abilities (and inabilities) and He knows just what you can and should do, for maximum weight loss results!

But ...to get all this "inside information" YOU HAVE TO ASK HIM! You have to purposely choose to include Him in this area of your life!

So...to make that happen, on this program, through this prayer, you are going to ask Him every day, to be your "Personal Trainer" so to speak.

You see, by asking the Holy Spirit every day to lead you in this way, He's on the scene! He'll be working hard to walk you down this path to health and fitness just like a human "personal trainer" would be -- and your job, is to work hard to hear Him and obey! Amen?

Let me remind you here, that Romans 8:14 tells us, that those that are "led by the spirit" are the sons of God!

And in case you didn't know that Greek word for "son" there, implies a level of maturity. In other words, not a "child" or a "baby" Christian, but a "son" or a "grown up" Christian. In fact the Passion translation, translates this verse like this:

### Romans 8:14 The Passion Translation

The mature children of God are those who are moved by the impulses of the Holy Spirit.

Church, what does this tell us? It tells us that IF, we want to be "mature" as God's children, then we are supposed to be moved / or "led" by the Holy Spirit!

*So why have we not been allowing the Holy Spirit to lead us in this aspect of our lives?*

Let me suggest, and I'm not meaning to sound judgmental here, but let me just throw this out as a theory. That IF. . . we are not listening to the leading of the Spirit in this area, could that imply, that we are not fully mature. . .. and that maybe, that's why we are having problems?

OUCH, right?

Look with me at this: This is out of the New King James version OPEN BIBLE, expanded edition, and it reads like this:

### Proverbs 30:8

. . .. Give me neither poverty nor riches,

Feed me with the food You prescribe for me. . ..

Church, this is out of the book of Proverbs, which is the book of wisdom!

Could it be, that we haven't been using wisdom in our eating because we haven't been listening to the Lord about what and how much to eat?

A prescription tells you "what" and "how much" of something to take, right?

Well, are we letting the Holy Spirit "prescribe" our food? He wants to, you know. And HE WILL. . . if you let Him!

Let me tell you a story.

Many years ago, my husband and I went to the Houston Open Golf Tournament. I was new at trying to listen to the Lord about my eating, but I was trying.

So we had been in 100-degree Texas heat all day, and had been just dripping with sweat, and as soon as we left and got on the road, we stopped at Whataburger. (It's a Texas thing!)

Now I was starving, but I was trying to listen to the Lord because I was just starting to work this "system" that I'm teaching you here, and I prayed really quick and asked the Lord what I should eat as I walked in. And as soon as I did, I knew the Lord spoke to my heart, to get a child's burger meal.

Now of course it was not audible words, it's just that I felt it really strong in my spirit that that's what He was prompting me to get.

And even though I KNEW that's what He was putting on my heart to order, I went up to the counter and out of my mouth came, "I'll have A double meat burger, with a large fry and large coke"

You see, I was starving and hadn't eaten all day and my "flesh" wanted a lot of food and wanted it NOW! So because I thought *I knew better than the Holy Spirit,* I just straight up ignored Him and I got myself, *what I felt* would be best.

Well, you can probably guess where this story is going. In my pride and my blatant disobedience, I ate my double meat burger, scarfing it down like a hungry dog. And then, about ten minutes later, it hit me. Ohhhhh....UGH! I had a terrible stomachache all the way home and when I got home, I threw up!

Now that's been years ago (and it's a really dumb story) but I have never forgotten it. Because here's the deal.

I was trying to train myself to listen to the Holy Spirit in my eating and even though I asked Him what to eat and, I felt like He answered, I purposely ignored it!

You see, because I had been so hot all day, He knew, my stomach couldn't handle that much food, and he knew, that a smaller meal would be enough to eat without getting sick. And if I just had obeyed. . . I would have been fine. ☹

So I say that not to say that if you don't obey the Holy Spirit you'll throw up, (ha-ha) but to say, what I'm telling you here, WORKS!

As mature Believers you know the voice of the Lord. But are you listening to His voice when it comes to your eating?

I want you to know that the Holy Spirit WILL lead you in your eating habits in absolutely incredible ways IF you will just ask Him to!

And, since He's going to be working with you to lose weight, you have to realize that His directions followed *will* produce supernatural weight loss results!

Now again, we'll talk more about the specifics of eating in another chapter, but for now, let's go on.

The next part of the prayer that you will be praying each day gets a little serious. But before I show you what you'll pray, let me explain the methodology behind it behind it first.

You see, on this program and through this prayer, you will, every day, with your words, "bless" your body.

But then, you will *also* every day, with your words, "curse" the extra weight on your body and command it to be removed and cast into the sea. We get this principle from this passage.

## <u>Mark 11:12-14, 20-23 New King James Version</u>

Now the next day, when they had come out from Bethany, He was hungry. And seeing from afar a fig tree having leaves, He went to see if perhaps He would find something on it. When He came to it, He found nothing but leaves, for it was not the season for figs. In response Jesus said to it, "Let no one eat fruit from you ever again." And His disciples heard it. . .

. . . Now in the morning, as they passed by, they saw the fig tree dried up from the roots. And Peter, remembering, said to Him, "Rabbi, look! The fig tree which You cursed has withered away." So Jesus answered and said to them, "Have faith in God. For assuredly, I say to you, whoever says to this mountain, 'Be removed and be cast into the sea,' and does not doubt in his heart, but believes that those things he says will be done, he will have whatever he says.

Now I want us to ponder on the principles we see within this text but first, I have a question.

How many times have we spoken word curses over our body in the midst of our weight loss struggles?

"I'm so fat!" "I'm gross!" "I'll never lose this weight!"

Friend, speaking that over ourselves is actually empowering all those spirits that we previously discussed and is keeping their influence strong in our lives!

Every time we come in agreement with the devil's plan to make and keep us overweight, we strengthen the hold of that extra weight on our body!

Every time we say something like, "I'm so fat…" or, "I *can't* lose weight", the bands of that invisible bondage get tighter!

Friend, you've got to decide right here and right now, that you are no longer going to speak in agreement with the devil's strategy for this area of your life!

I don't care how fat you feel, or how miserable you are, do not speak it out!  Do not insult your body, with your words, because that plays right into the enemy's hands!

You see, here's the bottom line.  It's **NOT** your body's fault!

Your body **WANTS TO BE** at a healthy weight!

And it's crying out for you to help it, to free it up, because the culprit here, is not your body.

It's the **EXTRA WEIGHT** on your body that is above and beyond God's will for you!

Therefore, at this point in the daily prayer that I'm about to show you, you are going to re-affirm to your body that you love it by taking the time to purposely bless your body!

Because whether you know it or not, the blessing you release from your spirit, with your words, contains tangible spiritual substance!

In fact, one definition of the blessing is, "the power to prosper".

So by blessing your body every day, you're going to "empower it to prosper", in each and every aspect of what you do to lose weight!

Now next, you will continue in the prayer, by speaking over and into your body and calling it "lean, strong and healthy". And I use that particular phrase because that's the phrase the Lord spoke to me years ago, when I first began seeking Him for revelation concerning this area of my life.

He said that anyone, of any bone structure and frame size, CAN BE "lean, strong and healthy" with His help!

Because remember, the purpose of this program is not to try to make us all "perfect". Believe me, I am far from perfect!

But, I do feel comfortable now and don't have all those mental hang-ups I once had in this area and that to me is a great blessing!

So I exhort you to simply make it your goal to BE and to FEEL, "lean, strong and healthy" for your particular body frame in this particular season of your life. Amen?

And I mention the "season" because our body weight and mass just natural changes throughout our lives, and we have to allow for that. You see not long ago I was talking to a lady in her 60's who told me her goal was to weigh what she weighed in high school. High School? Really? Guys... seasons change! Those days are long gone! Amen?

And maybe I'm wrong, but I highly doubt God is desiring for a mature woman of God to weigh what she did in high school. Because my gut tells me, that since that was like, 40 plus years ago...that may not be realistic!

So we need to understand, that all we need to be concerned with is, God's will for our body in THIS SEASON of our life. That's what I have trained myself to do and it's very freeing. Especially now, the older I get! (ha-ha)

In fact, truthfully, I don't even weigh myself anymore. Now I did when I started this journey years ago, but now, I go more by how my clothes fit and feel and if I can just throw something on and run out the door, without changing outfits 10 times to try to find something I don't look fat in!

Has anyone been there?

And I defend my position on weighing myself constantly by saying this.

The Bible says, on earth as it in in Heaven, right?

Well, to the best of my knowledge...there are no scales up in heaven. . . so why should I be concerned with scales here on earth? 😊

But look, I know that a lot of people do want to weigh themselves. And if that's you, that's fine. But let me suggest that if you do want to weigh yourself, you only do it ONCE A MONTH.

Why?

Because there are just too many ways the enemy can manipulate the scale! And you might feel like you're doing really good and be kind of proud of yourself, and then you weigh yourself, and if it doesn't say what *you think it should say,* then the devil's got you all upset! Amen?

You know my dear old mom used to have a saying. Every day, she would wake up and weigh herself. And she would say, "If I LOST a pound I'll be in a good mood . . . but if I GAINED a pound, I'll be in a bad mood!"

And really that contains a lot of truth, unfortunately, about how the scale can affect us.

I mean we are children of God! Why should we let a little metallic device with springs determine our mood for the day?

Now again, as with ALL of this, you do whatever you want!

But if I am "feeling" thinner and my clothes are loose, and I go to the store and have to buy a smaller size then that makes me happy! So to me, how I feel about myself is the better "barometer" of how the Lord is working in this area of my life!

Alrighty, so. . .let's move on!

By following this part of the prayer (which I'll show you in just a bit) you will next, attack the actual problem. And "the problem" is, THE EXTRA WEIGHT on your body that you and the Lord both know, shouldn't be there!

Remember church, your body is NOT the bad guy! The extra weight on your body is the bad guy! And THAT'S what you have to come against!

I like to look at it like this:

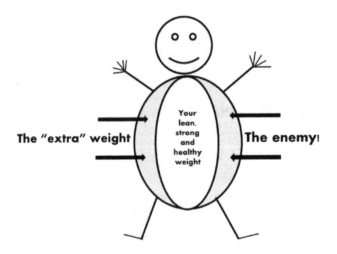

This is you, being lean strong and healthy. But, the extra weight that's not God's will for you IS ON TOP OF THAT (so to speak) and THAT'S what has to go!

And one of the first ways we are going to come against it, comes from that passage we just read.

If you remember in that passage it tells us that Jesus "cursed" the fig tree. He said it was "not producing fruit", so he used His words to evoke a curse into it and we read that it later, "withered away".

Well, here's the principle.

That extra weight on your body is "not producing fruit"! It is not "fruitful" for your health OR your self-esteem. It is not a positive, productive, beneficial thing for your life or your body. It has NO advantages, only disadvantages, because it causes you to be oppressed mentally, emotionally and physically, correct?

So if that's the case and that extra weight is only providing negative consequences, do you not think the Lord will agree with you if you want it to go? If you want that extra weight that is "weighing you down" to leave?

He has put supernatural power in your words, Believer. And while you do not want to curse YOUR BODY anymore, I believe you have every right and the power, to curse the mounds of useless adipose tissue that have made their home in, on and between the tissues and organs in your body.

Think of it this way. Those of us who know how to pray, know that when we are praying for folks, who have say, tumors or cysts and/or growths in their bodies, that we pray AGAINST those things, right? As a mature Believer, if someone came to us and said, they had some sort of "growth" beginning to show up on their body, what would we do?

We would "CURSE" that tumor or growth at the root, right? And we would command it to wither and leave their bodies, correct?

Well, this is the exact same principle that you'll use in this part of the prayer! Only you'll be praying over YOURSELF and cursing that useless, extra FAT! Amen?

So... having said all of that, let me show you now, this part of the prayer that you will pray every day.

This paragraph of the Power Prayer reads like this. You'll say:

*I bless my body today Lord, and call it lean, strong and healthy..... but I curse the extra weight on my body and command it to "be removed and cast into the sea"!*

See, you are "blessing" your body, because you love your body and you want it to be blessed, right? And then you are using your words, to speak forth into existence what you desire, by calling it "lean, strong and healthy", amen?

But *then...* you'll say, "I CURSE the extra weight on my body" ( because remember it's nothing but a hindrance) and you'll command it to "be removed" and "cast into the sea" just like Jesus taught us, amen?

I mean, didn't Jesus say, "speak to the mountain and command it to be removed"? Well that "mountain of extra weight" is going to be SHOCKED when you start talking to it!

It's been laying there happily taking over your body and it's not going to believe that you know now that you can speak to it and command it to be removed! ☺

I'm telling you your words of blessings and curses have power friend! You were made in the image of God and God speaks things into existence and so can you!

You, blessing your body, is going to make your body SO happy!

And, that extra fat is going to begin to break down SUPERNATURALLY, because you are cursing it and commanding it to go in Jesus' name! Yay, yay, yay!

Ok now. . . let's move on!

In the next part of the prayer we will begin to tap into another "supernatural" part of this plan.

You see friend, I believe the reason so many of us have weight problems, and the reason so many of us can't seem to lose weight, is because we have tried to depend too much on our OWN efforts when it comes to weight loss.

It's our food, our mouth, our body, so we just figure it's our problem to deal with on our own, right? Wrong!

Don't we know that as long as we fight ANY battle with our own strength, we will never defeat our enemy? 2 Corinthians 10:4 says, "the weapons of our warfare are not carnal. . .but mighty through God for the pulling down of strongholds."

Meaning. . .

the weapons WE as Christians are to use to fight our battles are not to be "carnal", or just of our human efforts -- they are to be weapons that are "mighty through God" because that's what will pull down the strongholds! Amen?

So again, why are fighting THIS battle, our "weight battle" with our human strength alone?

Public Service Announcement: THAT'S BEEN THE PROBLEM!

We've been fighting this weight battle with carnal weapons instead of spiritual weapons!

We haven't been "warfaring" the extra weight...we've just been dieting and exercising and "doing stuff" that we thought would make us lose weight through our own human efforts!

However, and now get this. . . when we fight our weight battle THROUGH THE SPIRIT REALM FIRST, it becomes a whole new game!

Friends, we need God's strength for this battle!

We need the supernatural power of the Holy Spirit that we know, can make the blind see, the deaf hear, and the dead live again! We need miraculous, supernatural, Holy Ghost, wonder working power to get this weight off and it's time we start to tap into it in a mighty way!

You know I don't know if you realize this, but there are people involved in occultic practices on this earth who take their craft very, very, seriously. They do all sorts of rituals and make sacrifices and pray and chant for hours to tap into demonic strength. And their diligence, to the ways of the ENEMY, causes them to be "supernaturally indwelt" with the devil's power. Then with that power they do many evil, supernatural things, usually to bring harm to others or to territories or regions.

Church WAKE UP!

Don't we know that anything the enemy's camp does is simply a counterfeit copy of a spiritual truth found in God's Kingdom?

Then here's what we can learn from this.

These people spend CONCENTRATED EFFORT, and purposely USE THEIR TIME doing things to GAIN DEMONIC SPIRITUAL POWER.

While, for the most part, "the church", is TOO APATHETIC AND DISTRACTED, TO SPEND THE TIME NEEDED TO HAVE GOD'S POWER IN AND ON OUR LIVES!

And I don't mean to be fussing at you, I'm just hoping to light a fire in your heart! Because I want you to know that if you really focus on this and pray the daily Power Prayer with belief and determination and get deadly serious, about not only praying forth God's power, but about working WITH that power, you will see change!

*Supernatural, miraculous change!*

And when people say to you, "dang, you have really lost some weight!" You will be able to say, "Praise God! The Lord did this for me!" Amen? Because friend, that's what it's ultimately all about! Giving Him Glory in and through our lives!

So let me close this chapter by telling you this.

Right now. . . at this very second... YOU HAVE THE POWER AVAILABLE TO YOU TO BECOME LEAN, STRONG AND HEALTHY FOR THE GLORY OF GOD! IF.... YOU'LL SIMPLY TAKE THE TIME TO MAKE IT WORK!

In fact, truthfully, I am begging you to decide right now, that you are going to take on a dominion attitude here! A warrior type mindset! And then, begin to come against the extra weight on your body, seeing it as THE ENEMY to your health and self-esteem that it is!

Friend, I'm tired of Believers dying prematurely! How many mighty destinies have been thwarted because the carrier of that destiny had obesity related problems with their health?

It's time for us to "rule and reign" in this area like the Kingly, Royal powerful children of God that we are!

Can you get on board with that? Do you not know that our God is greater than any obstacle on the earth? And He is SURE greater than the blobs of extra adipose tissue lying dormant all over your body!

But you've got to believe that! And then you've got to get mad as heck at the devil, who's been playing you all these years and get "all in" dedicated to praying forth and working with God's power, as you drive the extra weight off of your body and out of your life!

So are you fired up yet? I hope so, because now I want to explain to you the power that you'll be tapping into. ( Drumroll please. . . .)

It's the anointing power of the Holy Spirit! Which is, God's supernatural power in and on your life!

Look with me at this:

### Isaiah 10:27 New King James Version
It shall come to pass in that day
That his burden will be taken away from your shoulder,
And his yoke from your neck,
And the yoke will be destroyed because of the anointing.

Friends, **GOD'S ANOINTING** on you in the various ways we are about to discuss is what will "remove the burden" and "destroy the yoke" of the extra weight on your body! And what you're about to discover is that receiving God's Anointing daily has been the missing key!

# THE ANOINTING

In the last chapter we looked at Isaiah 10:27. This verse tells us that the Anointing "removes burdens and destroys yokes, correct?

Well, would you not agree with me that that extra weight on your body is a "burden" *and* a "yoke"?

Ok then if that's so (and it is!) then what I need you to understand today is that the Anointing is the secret to removing that extra weight!

Now you may think that sounds crazy, or even sacrilegious! But I assure you it's not. You see, tapping into the anointing is a huge piece of this puzzle, so please don't think that the Lord wouldn't want to "waste" His Anointing on something as trivial as your weight problem. If the devil is putting that lie into your mind, let me just remind you of this.

Friend, the care of and the good stewardship of your body is a big deal to God! According to 1 Corinthians 6:19, your body is

## God's TEMPLE!

You see, it really doesn't even belong to you. It belongs to Him. Because as a Believer, it's where He dwells. So the care of your body, HIS temple, is in fact, extremely important in God's eyes!

And too you have to remember, that your body is the only vehicle you have to carry your spirit! And it's the only means you have of doing the work of the Kingdom that God has ordained you to do while you are on the earth!

So the point I am trying to make is that as Christians, we've got to stop being so apathetic about the care of our body. We've got to stop being so careless and irresponsible, because we only get ONE BODY in life. . . and once it ceases to function, and we die, we will stand before God and give an account of our life. And if we had years and years of our calling to still complete, that we were NOT able to fulfill because we ate too much and we exercised too little, there will be no going back. There will be no "do- overs". Once we die, we're dead. It's over! So we need to realize right here and now, that the care of our bodies....the good "stewardship" of *His* temple. . . GREATLY matters to God!

Have you ever really thought about it like that?

Most of us haven't.

And who do you think would want us NOT to think this subject through this way? The devil and his cohorts, that's who!

Why?

Because as long as you don't get focused on this. . . as long as you stay too busy, or too tired, or continue to believe that the care of your body really isn't a big deal to God, then by default, the enemy will come in with all little schemes to do whatever he can to put you in a state of bad health!

Let me show you that analogy in the Word.

### Proverbs 24:30-34 Easy-to-Read Version

I walked past a field that belonged to a lazy man.
It was a vineyard that belonged to someone who understood
nothing.
Weeds were growing everywhere!
Wild vines covered the ground, and the wall around the
vineyard was broken and falling down.


I looked at this and thought about it. This is what I learned:
a little sleep, a little rest, folding your arms, and taking a nap—
these things will make you poor very quickly.
Soon you will have nothing, as if a thief broke in and took
everything away.



Can you see the point within this proverb? We live in a sin cursed world. So anything we remain ignorant of, anything we just leave alone, don't take care of, or ignore, will deteriorate! It will get weak and damaged, because *unless there is definite positive action put towards the taking care of that thing, the curse of sin will remain unopposed and the destruction of it will be the result!*

Well let's apply that truth to the care of our bodies. And then, let's add in what I'm sharing with you here.

Church, the Anointing IS and HAS BEEN the missing ingredient in our weight struggles!

And once you start to pray forth the Anointing (by following the next section of the prayer that I'm about to show you) THE POWER IS THERE! The power of God to actively work AGAINST the curse of sin operating in your body is there! Because through the Anointing, every aspect of what you will need to eat right, exercise and lose weight, will be IN YOU and ON YOU to walk in a "weight loss lifestyle" for the rest of your life!

I'm telling you friend, it's so crazy good!

Once you start to pray forth the Anointing, you do things that are "weight loss friendly", that you never wanted to do before!

And you'll find yourself saying things such as, "I can't believe I don't even want that second helping" . . . or, "I can't believe I walked for a whole hour and didn't get winded" . . . or, "I can't believe these jeans are lose, they've been skintight for the last 10 years!" (Ha-ha)

I'm telling you church, THIS WORKS!

The Anointing is God's invisible power that empowers you in whatever way you pray it forth! And, when you start to pray it forth in the ways I'm about to show you, everything comes together in your life to make you lose the extra weight!

So with all that said, let's jump right in and I'll explain to you the various anointings you'll be praying forth. And then, I'll show you how it fits into the Daily Prayer.

The first Anointing you will pray forth is what I call the anointing of "weight loss". That sounds reasonable enough in this context, right? But is there an anointing for that in the Word? I'm glad you asked! Look with me at this:

### Isaiah 10:16 New King James Version

Therefore the Lord, the Lord of hosts,
Will send leanness among his fat ones. . .

Ohhhh K! Well, here's the deal!

That Hebrew word for "leanness" there, is the word "Razown".

It is defined as "a wasting away of, a decrease in measure, or thinness" and it's derived from the root word "razah" which means "to make or become thin"!

Now what I want you to grasp today, is that in this verse, we see the Lord releasing "leanness", which means thinness! He was releasing His power to make their bodies lean / thin!

Can you catch the magnitude of that?

Please see this. It says in verse 16, He will SEND. . . "leanness", which is the Hebrew word for THINNESS!

So what does that say to us?  It tells us that our God, has the power within him, that can be released to make a body thin!

Can you believe it?  It's true!

You've got to get this today my friend!  GOD'S POWER WAS GOING INTO THEIR BODIES AND SHRINKING THEM! It was making them decrease in size!  IT WAS MAKING THEM THINNER. . . and this is also what He can do for YOU!

I really need you to take hold of the fact that the Word shows us this attribute of God!  Because if God has it, then WE can ask for it!  And He has it -- because we see it being released from Him in this verse!

Now let me interject here, a little explanation about this before

64

we go on. You see in the context of this verse, he was releasing this "razown" -- this "leanness" / thinness, into the Assyrian army as a negative thing because they were the enemies of Israel.

So in the context of this verse in Isaiah, please understand that it was a NOT a "happy go lucky" weight loss thing. Because this power was being used by God to bring judgment upon them so that they would die! Yipes!

Also, let interject here too, that a lot of Bible versions translate this word into the term, "a wasting disease". But that's not what it was!

It was acting like a wasting disease would... because it was shrinking their bodies and decreasing their body weight. . . just like how an extremely sick person would just "waste away". But if you study it out, it wasn't a disease! God does not have disease in Him to release! No, it was this Hebrew word, razown, which means TO MAKE THIN!

Now, with all with that said, let's think for minute about how this can relate to your weight struggles.

Friend, we have a God who has this power! Let me repeat that so I know you understand.

As a born-again Believer, YOU HAVE A GOD WHO HAS WITHIN HIM THE POWER TO MAKE A BODY THIN!

And although in the context of this passage He was releasing it into them as punishment, the truth of the matter is that we see here that this specific dimension of God's power exists!

God has the power of "leanness" church! The power of "thinness"! In other words, God has the power to make you lose weight!

Therefore, for simplicity sake, that's what we are going to call this Anointing! We will refer to the power we see in this verse as, the "Anointing to lose weight", because all I really need you to understand here is that this power is real!

The power to make you become "lean" . . . to literally SHRINK your body, like it did to the Assyrians, is real! It's in God's Omnipotence! And it's available to you IF you will just pray it forth!

Sooooo. . . on this program, you will be directed to pray forth this anointing every morning by following the Power Prayer. And this part of the prayer looks like this.

*I receive your Anointing for weight loss today Lord, and I decree that I am lean in Jesus' name!*

Now I want you to notice what you'll be doing here.

For the various Anointings I am about to explain to you, you simply will each day, **PURPOSELY** receive them. Because believe it or not, purposely "receiving" is an especially important spiritual action and one that we don't talk about near enough!

Think about it. When you "received" Jesus as your personal Savior, that salvation was "out there" in the invisible spirit realm available to you, but it didn't become yours.... until you **CHOSE** to purposely "receive" it. Right?

And let's take this one step further. When you received Jesus as your Savior, think about the movement in the Spirit realm that took place. He went from being "out there" (in the atmosphere so to speak) to being, "in here" (inside of your now born-again spirit)!

When you said, "Jesus I **RECEIVE** you as my Savoir", you caused movement to happen! He tangibly moved, from "out there" to "in here", to reside inside your spirit.

So I said all that to get you to understand the importance of receiving these anointings every day.

When you say, "I receive your Anointing for weight loss" . . . **THE POWER OF THE HOLY SPIRIT FOR WEIGHT LOSS IS ACTIVATED AND IT THEN MOVES INTO AND ONTO YOUR BODY!**

It's there! Your words, your faith, and you purposely

**RECEIVING IT,** pulls it out of God's invisible realm of power and places it upon you for that day!

Isn't that amazing?

And let me add one more thing before we go on. As we pray forth all these anointings, you will then, make a decree, as to what you are believing that anointing to do.

Now, as mature believers, I'm sure you know the power of a decree, so I won't teach you that. But I want you to see on this one, how this goes. You'll say:

*"I receive your Anointing for Weight Loss today Lord,*

(now remember this is that Hebrew word defined as "leanness" that we saw in Isaiah 10, but we are just putting it in an easy to relate to term) but then you'll say, "and I decree that I am lean in Jesus' name"!

You see, you will receive the Anointing. . . and then, speak into the Anointing a decree of what you are desiring it to do!

And you'll do this with each aspect of the Anointing we are about to discuss, but don't let this confuse you right now. You're smart, mature Believers, so I promise it will all come together in the end! 😊

Let's move on.

The next Anointing we will be praying forth each day is the

anointing of self-control. Look with me at this.

### Galatians 5:22-23 (New King James Version)

But the fruit of the Spirit is love, joy, peace, patience, kindness, goodness, faithfulness, gentleness and self-control.

We see here that "self-control" is part of the Fruit of the Spirit that we are exhorted to walk in in Galatians 5. So the truth of the matter is, that we are supposed to be walking in it. . . but how many of us really are?

Well, by praying forth the "anointing of self-control" . . .God's very own empowerment for self-control, guess what? You will, supernaturally, through the natural, begin to exhibit supernatural self- control in your eating and exercise habits! Isn't' that exciting! Praise the Lord!

Now let me show you something.

### Titus 2:1-2 The Passion Translation

Your duty is to teach them to embrace a lifestyle that is consistent with sound doctrine. [2] Lead the elders into disciplined lives full of dignity and self-control. Urge them to have a solid faith, generous love, and patient endurance.

In this passage, the Apostle Paul is expressing to Titus the character traits consistent with the spiritual maturity needing to be expressed by Christian leaders. And we see here that self-control is a part of that list.

So what does that tell us?

It tells us that if we desire to be truly Christlike . . . and if we desire to be in a position of spiritual leadership, self-control is supposed to be an irrefutable character trait in our life!

So intercessors, prayer warriors and mature Believers, let me exhort you to stop and really self -examine yourself here. Because it's time for us to get serious about this issue, and show the people who look up to us, how a disciplined, mature, self- controlled Believer should act!

You see, we preach about the Fruit of the Spirit... and we tell our people, we need to control our tongues......control our anger....and control our gossip. . . (in other words, we are to control what comes OUT of our mouths) but why do we not stress this trait when it comes to what we put IN our mouths?

And I'm not talking about being legalistic or rude about it, or, being full of condemnation. I'm just saying that as spiritual leaders, why do we preach, teach and tell others that we are supposed to be self-controlled in other areas, but when it comes to HOW MUCH WE EAT, we never plug into our own advice?

Now please remember that picture I showed earlier when I weighed almost 100 pounds more than I do now. I was teaching 2 Bible studies a week at this time! I was a youth pastor and teaching a class called "POWER DISCIPLESHIP"! So I promise I am NOT trying to make you feel bad! Nor, am I trying to act super-spiritual! But please friend, let the Holy Spirit convict you if need be!

Because sometimes, it's not until we truly, truly see that we *need* to change, that the change will come forth! Amen?

And look, self-control is a hard one for all of us.

But if we really ponder on it, it truly is a "make it" or "break it" quality in the Christian life! I mean if you don't use self-control...you could end up in jail! Amen?

And think about the ramifications that a lack of self - control had in the life of Adam.

The fall of mankind, the loss of the Glory covering and the entering in of the curse upon the entire earth. . . ALL CAME ABOUT, essentially because Adam did not use self-control!

So could we be hurting our OWN lives in various ways because we are not using self-control in some areas where we should? Definitely something to think about, amen?

You see, we can't "pick and choose" the activities in which we are going to express spiritual maturity. It's like that joke that says, "How many pushups can Chuck Norris do?"  Answer: ALL OF THEM!

Well church, what we need to take ownership of, is the fact that we are called to walk in ALL of these traits, in EVERY AREA of our life. Including in our eating!

Which we will begin to do as we start praying the prayer! Yay!

So, with all that said, let me show you now, this section of the prayer. It reads like this.

*I receive your Anointing of Self-Control today and I decree that I eat ONLY what and how much you direct me to eat in Jesus' name!*

Ok, at this point, I would like to interject a few things about this decree before we continue.

As you see, after you pray and purposely receive God's Anointing for Self-control every day, you will say, "I decree I eat ONLY what and how much you direct me to eat in Jesus' name!"

Let me explain.

Earlier in the prayer, you asked the Holy Spirit to "lead, guide and direct you" in your eating habits. And because you have asked for this, He will indeed do just that! (Remember my

Whataburger story?)

Yes, be assured, HE is going to do his part!   So your part, is to simply OBEY!

Meaning, simply eat whatever the Lord tells/ directs/ prompts/ leads you to eat. . .  and be careful too, to obey his directions as to how much!

Now truthfully, this will probably be similar, yet different for all of us!

He may put it on your heart to follow a low-calorie, or low carbohydrate meal plan. Or, He may prompt you to follow a "Weight Watchers" or a "Keto" type of eating strategy.

You see, since there are all sorts of programs and eating plans out there, He may know that **FOR YOU**, it would just be easier for you to follow something that is already planned out.

Now personally, I don't think God advocates any particular program, because the program is not your power source here. Being led by the Holy Spirit is your "power source".

However, because He knows you so well, He may know, that a pre-set type of meal plan is what would work easiest and most effectively in your life.  I don't know your particulars, but I know the bottom line is this; **JUST SEEK HIM ABOUT THIS AND FOLLOW HIS LEAD!**

Ask Him to show you and then do some research to try to determine how He is leading you.

Do you know that the Holy Spirit sometimes speaks through natural information? Get on the computer and ask Him to lead you as you search out a viable and workable eating strategy. Or, maybe just ask around.

Find out what's working for people you know. Find out what's available and able to fit into your particular lifestyle and within your financial budget.

If you ask Him to show you how HE wants you to eat and then study out your options, I promise you He won't ignore your request.

Also, let me add a reminder that He is not a cruel taskmaster!

His yoke is easy, and His burden is light, right? He's NOT going to starve you to death, and He WILL allow for special occasions and Holidays without condemnation and guilt. He loves you! He wants you to enjoy food and life, He just wants you to always be following His lead!

In fact, let me take a minute and throw this theory out there.

Do you realize that one of God's very first instructions to man was about his eating? Look with me at this.

## Genesis 2:16-17 New King James Version

And the LORD God commanded the man, saying, "Of every tree of the garden you may freely eat; but of the tree of the knowledge of good and evil you shall not eat, for in the day that you eat of it you shall surely die.

Here we see very clearly that God directed, well, He actually "commanded", man as to WHAT HE COULD EAT and what he was NOT TO EAT. So why would we think He wouldn't want to do the same to us today?

Well guess what? He does and He will! If we will just allow Him to! And by doing so, I promise you it will prove to be extremely beneficial to your life! Now I mentioned this earlier, but let me remind you of this verse again:

## 2 Corinthians 3:17 (New International Version)

Now the Lord is the Spirit, and where the Spirit of the Lord is, there is freedom.

Church, if we are overweight and miserable about it, we are in bondage! And what is the opposite of bondage? FREEDOM, right?

Well friend, that is exactly what the Holy Spirit brings!

So get this: **IF YOU ALLOW THE HOLY SPIRIT TO DIRECT YOU IN YOUR EATING, HE WILL BRING YOU TO A PLACE OF FREEDOM IN THIS AREA OF YOUR LIFE!**

It's what He does. . . and it's what He is!

So why do we not include Him in this?  I mean think about it. We eat, pretty much all day long, every single day of our life!

Why would we think that this is **NOT** something that He wants to direct?

I feel we have been so blinded in this area!

It's like we for the most part, have made the Lord the Lord of **EVERY** part of our lives, except **THIS** part!  And then we wonder why the majority of us are overweight!

Friends, I have been following this principle for many years now and I promise you the Holy Spirit **WILL** indeed lead you in your eating habits if you give Him the chance.

But for now, let's go back to the specifics, and let me explain this.

Like I said, the Holy Spirit **MAY** lead you to follow some type of pre-set eating plan.  **OR**. . . He may lead you to just kind of create your own eating strategy out of various plans you may have used or been familiar with before.

Now, for me, personally, at this point in my journey, I don't feel led to follow any pre-set meal plans or systems and you may not either. What I do now is, simply take it on a **MEAL-BY-MEAL BASIS** and just listen to the Lord, concerning each individual meal or snack.

And by that I mean, that I will simply take in account whatever I have available, either at home or, from selections at a restaurant, and pray about what the choices are for me from out of that.

Which means I pretty much just say before I choose, "What do you want me to eat for (breakfast ... or lunch... or dinner) Holy Spirit?"

And then I'll just ponder on that and go with what I feel in my heart, and have peace about, eating for that meal.

But let me add this.

When you first start this weight loss battle, Holy Spirit may make things a bit more restrictive for a while. Which means you may feel led to eat a low calorie, or a low carbohydrate diet for a season or, He may lead you to fast in some form for a certain period of time to get a good strong weight loss start!

For instance, He may put it on your heart to fast from dinner for the first 21 days or something similar to that. Or, He may put it on your heart to only have a Protein Shake for breakfast and dinner for a while, but to have a big healthy filling lunch.

I don't know your specifics and am just using these as

examples, because the Holy Spirit's instructions will be different for everyone. But He has led me to do that type thing before, in which I felt His prompting to substitute some of my meals with Protein shakes. And we will talk more about that in a bit, but for now, let me finish up this chapter with a few more suggestions.

First of all, let me suggest that when you decide to start this program, that you clean out your pantry of the "junk foods". I'm sure you know what they are and, that you know deep down inside of you somewhere that they really shouldn't be there.

Because I need you to realize from this time on, that those high fat, high sugar junk foods, have been "tools" that the enemy has been using to keep you in bondage!

You see, if you don't put some sort of negative connotation on that stuff, the enemy is going to tell you, "you paid good money for those twinkies, don't throw them away. . . there are starving children in China don't ya know?"

Yeah. . . he'll put whatever thought in your head he can to get you to hang on to his temptations! But I want you to see yourself like Adam and Eve. What IF...they had taken that forbidden fruit and thrown it in the garbage? We wouldn't be in the mess we are in today, right? (Ha-ha!)

Guys, you can do this! A new start requires some new actions! And sometimes you have to get rid of the OLD to allow the

NEW to come in! Amen?

If throwing away that junk food seems like a lot to ask, let me assure you of this.

Once you start praying this way every day, YOUR MINDSET AND YOUR TASTE PREFERENCES ARE GOING TO SUPERNATURALLY CHANGE!

I telling you, it's true! Once you start to ask the Holy Spirit to help you, that candy bar and Dr. Pepper you HAD to have every afternoon is NOT going to taste good anymore! It just won't!

And that fatty Bacon Burger you used to always grab in the drive through, is going to make you feel miserable and YOU JUST WON'T WANT IT ANYMORE! And when you stop to think about why you feel this way, there won't be any *natural* explanation for it at all!

And it isn't that the Holy Spirit is being harsh towards you, He's not!

He loves you and wants what's best for you. So He'll be working supernaturally, through the natural, to make you NOT want the stuff the enemy used to tempt you with, but instead, He'll cause you to WANT what He knows will make you lean, strong and healthy from here on out! Yay!

So once you make that food "closet cleanout" and you pray and get some directions from the Lord on how He wants you to eat, then next, it's time to replace that junk with some good, healthy stuff!

You know, salad fixings, fish and chicken, lots of fruit and green vegetables, etc. etc., etc....

Because while the Holy Spirit CAN work with "fast food" due to the world we live in, it's great to have some good healthy, lean, choices to grab for your dinner or to pack for lunch.

You see church, it's really easy to pick up on His promptings if you're just listening. And once you start to pray the daily prayer, you're spiritual ears will be opened to pick it all up!

Now we're going to talk a lot more about food choices in our next chapter but for now, let me finish this topic.

I want to suggest one more thing.

As you start this plan, get yourself a little notebook that you'll be able to keep with you throughout the day. It may have a calendar, or maybe not (you can always write the date at the top of the page) but make it something you can use to keep track of all you eat and if you exercise that day.

Having a "food journal" has been proven to help keep you focused. And, it's a really good way to start until all this becomes second nature to you, which I promise you it will!

So as we close this chapter, let me remind you of what Mary said to Jesus' servants at the wedding of Cana in John chapter two.

They had run out of wine and Mary went to Jesus to fix the problem. And if you remember the story, He hesitated at first, but then Mary looked at the servants and said, "Whatever He says to you, do it!"

Well I'm sure you know what happened next. Because they obeyed Jesus' directions, they had a MIRACULOUS CONVERSION of water turning into wine!

So let's be honest here. How many of us need a "miraculous conversion" in our bodies? Then here's my word to you today. Whatever He says to you do it!

Friend, the Lord's directions obeyed always produces miracles! So I want you to know that your obedience to His directions *concerning your eating habits* will, likewise, produce supernatural results! Amen? Amen!

# THE POWER OF PROTEIN

Let's now continue right where we left off in the previous chapter. If you remember, we were going over the section of the Daily Prayer, that says this:

*I receive your Anointing of Self-Control today and I decree that I eat only what and how much you direct me to eat in Jesus' name!*

Let's look again at the decree.

I want you to notice that after praying forth the Anointing, you're going decree that you "eat only what and how much you direct me to eat in Jesus name"!

You see, because you make this decree, that Anointing for self-control is going to be directed specifically towards you being "self-controlled" enough to obey the Holy Spirit and to eat only what you feel the Holy Spirit directs you to eat AND the amount.

And you may be reading this and thinking, "but how will I know what the Spirit directs me to eat?" And my answer to that is this. YOU'LL HAVE PEACE!

Look with me at this verse. It's Colossians 3:15, but it's out of the Good News Translation Bible because I love the way it reads. It says this:

<u>Colossians 3:15 Good News Translation</u>
The peace that Christ gives is to guide you in the decisions you make.

Isn't that powerful? Let's soak that up!

The PEACE that Christ gives, is to GUIDE YOU in the decisions you make! Friend, that includes the decisions you make as to what and how much you should eat!

Let me give you a pretend scenario example.

Let's say you get up in the morning and say your Daily Prayer. Then you go in the kitchen to eat breakfast.

So now, *before* you just grab something... or eat something simply out of habit. . . "well I always have a bowl of cereal" (or whatever) . . .

Yes, before you choose what you're going to eat, STOP. . . and ask the Holy Spirit, "What do YOU want me to have for Breakfast, Lord"?

Then, just take a few seconds, and think. . . and listen to your spirit.

Now I know you guys know how to hear the Lord, so I won't go into a big, detailed explanation about that. Because the hard part is just doing it! Just stopping long enough to *ask Him* and then, waiting for a second or two until you feel you get a response!

So now, let's say you stop before you eat and ask Him, and then it comes into your mind to have a protein shake, or some eggs, or whatever.

So when that thought comes up from your spirit. . . into your mind. . . you just go with it and have that!

It doesn't matter if that's not what you usually have.

If THAT'S what you feel like the Lord said when you asked Him, then, THAT'S what you are supposed to eat!

So then let's say, you felt led to eat whatever it may have been, then here's how you know if you heard Him and obeyed.

If you eat, what you felt like the Lord directed you to eat, then afterwards, you will just have peace!

You'll just feel sort of "proud" of yourself! Because you know that you asked, and you felt like you heard Him and obeyed what YOU BELIEVE He said to do!

And in your heart, you're just be like, "Yes! THAT'S what I was supposed to eat!" "It may not have been what I *wanted* to eat, but I believe that I obeyed, so yay me!" 😊

Now let me give you another scenario.

Let's say you woke up, said your daily prayer and go into the kitchen. But someone brought in a box of fresh, hot donuts!

And you look at them and with **NO THOUGHT AT ALL**, you grab one, eat it and realize it was soooo good, that you'll have another one. So you eat it too!

Then, you go to get ready for your day and you look down at your bedside table and see your daily prayer.

How are you going to feel, concerning what you just did?

You see friend, I'm not trying to shame you. I'm really not! I just want the Body of Christ to begin to be aware of this powerful trick of the enemy!

**THE DEVIL DOES NOT WANT YOU TO THINK ABOUT YOUR EATING!**

He just wants you to **MINDLESSLY STICK TERRIBLE FOOD IN YOUR MOUTH**, and not think about what you've done until the consequences of those choices appear in your life!

So let's say you just mindlessly woofed down 2 donuts simply because they were there. You can ignore it... or... if you stop and think it though.... and realize that you didn't even *think* about asking the Holy Spirit about eating them, you're going to feel a bit "convicted". Which means, you *won't* feel very proud of yourself, or have peace about that decision. Amen?

But let me interject here, that when that happens. . . and it will... you just repent and ask forgiveness and go on! You'll do better the next time, I promise!

You see on this plan, I want to exhort you and hopefully convince you, of the need to **STOP BEFORE YOU EAT AND ASK THE HOLY SPIRIT!** That's really all I am talking about here!

Now sometimes, the Lord *will* give you the green light to eat a donut, or a piece of cake or pie or something yummy. ( But remember to consult Him as to how much!) And realize too, He's not mean! He is just a genius weight loss strategist, that you are now supposed to be working with, because you have prayed His guidance in this area forth!

I mean think about it. If you hired a personal dietician and paid them tons of money to tell you how to eat, would you ignore what they said and do your own thing? No!

Well you've "hired" the Holy Spirit so to speak, by asking him to "lead, guide and direct you". So now, He's doing what you asked, but you have to do your part as well!

So, back to our donuts! When you see the donuts, just ask Him. And if you feel like He is giving you the "green light" then have one. ( Because I bet ONE is all He'll prompt you to have. . . ) But hey, enjoy it! Because if you've ASKED HIM FIRST and you felt like it was ok, then even after having a donut, you will still have peace! Because you know He loves you and while He wants you to enjoy life. . . He just wants to lead and direct you in this area. Amen?

Let me show you this:

### 1 Samuel 15:22 Easy-to-Read Version

But Samuel answered, "Which pleases the LORD more: burnt offerings and sacrifices or obeying his commands? It is better to obey the LORD than to offer sacrifices to him. It is better to listen to him than to offer the fat from rams.

Church, what are we going to do with that? It's right there! For us to listen to Him and just obey is what He truly wants!

And my theory is, why, oh why, are we not teaching this in our churches? It's not like eating is some little, tiny thing that we barely ever do! We eat, for the most part, all day long, every single day of our life!

*So why have we not been applying Biblical principles to our eating?*

Not religious, legalistic stuff, but practical spiritual principles that can help prevent us from getting into bondage in this area before it's too late!

And think about this. As Believers, why do we advise each other saying things such as, "Oh, you need to *pray about* what car to buy, you need to *pray about* where to live, you need to *pray about* who to date, etc., but we never bring that same "pray and seek the Lord first" mindset, into our eating? *The thing we do more than any other activity in our life?*

But anyway...now you know. Which is good, but bad. Because now you will be accountable for knowing it. But, I promise you, it's easy once you start doing it. And when you begin to see the supernatural results, you'll never stop! 😊

Okkkk. . . . having said all of that, I want to turn a corner here, and give you some straight up, "natural" teaching. In other words, some practical, real life, "biology/chemistry stuff" that we as Believers need to know!

You see friend, God is Spirit. And, He is invisible. And while yes, or course, He works according to His spiritual principles, most of the time He has to have natural vehicles to work His Spiritual principles through!

For instance, if you are praying for a certain bill to be paid, more often than not, he doesn't just go into the computer of the company and supernaturally make the bill say, "Paid in full", right?  Now He could. . . but most of the time, He'll work *through* some natural, real life vessel, to cause the money to pay the bill to be put in your hands.  And then YOU go pay the bill off. Correct?

So let's think this through. Because you prayed for the bill to be paid, and He miraculously got money to you, so that YOU could pay the bill, did God do it supernaturally? Yes!

But he used YOU. . . COOPERATING WITH CIRCUMSTANCES IN THE NATURAL REALM, to get it done!  Amen?

So, let's put that in the context of weight loss.

I know, beyond a shadow of a doubt, that the Lord is going to cause people who read this book or listen to this teaching (the live seminar is available as a series of videos at www.WarfareTheWeight.com) to supernaturally and miraculously lose weight!

I've already had testimonies of this happening, but the Lord has told me that some people are going to read the book, or watch the teaching, and just wake up the next morning, 5, 10, maybe 20 pounds lighter!

You see, I've been studying this subject for many years and the Lord has promised me that *that* was what He was going to do!

So praise the Lord!  That is going to be amazing and fun!

However...

I think the *majority* of the supernatural weight loss that is going to happen to those hearing this information will occur the other way. Supernaturally through the natural!

And because that's so, my thought is, that WE NEED TO HAVE ALL THE NATURAL KNOWLEDGE WE CAN GET ABOUT HOW OUR BODY WORKS AND WHAT CAUSES IT TO LOSE WEIGHT!

You see, I feel for the most part, that God works best...when we give him natural situations that are in agreement with, what we are asking Him to do.

Which means, if we are asking the Lord for the "weight loss anointing", we can't then, be sitting around on the couch all night eating cookies and ice cream!

We have to work WITH what we are ASKING HIM FOR and NOT AGAINST IT! Amen?

So with all that said, let's have a "Weight loss 101" class to cover all the things in the natural realm that we need to know. Because having this knowledge will enable us to produce with our actions, a weight loss friendly lifestyle that the Lord can bless!

But before I start, I want to make this disclaimer.

I am not a medical doctor and am not attempting to give medical or nutritional advice.

Any suggestions, tips and tricks that I share in this book are simply my sharing things I have done, and I am not instructing you to take, use, or ingest any specific foods or supplements.

I advise you as the reader, to consult your personal physician before making any changes in your diet or your supplementation habits.

So let me re-emphasis, that I am just going to share some of the things that I use and take. And I know that everyone's body is different, and that people have different health issues and take different medicines. So please check with your doctor and of course pray about all of this. And then, use any, all, of none of it, to work with the Holy Spirit to create an eating and supplement plan that is right for you!

You see, I'm simply advising you to have your spiritual ears open, and if some of the things I share speak to your spirit, then look into them and pray about if the Lord is recommending them for you too.

Now, I want to start this part by sharing with you some basic physiological facts about how God made our body to work.

This is super simplified, and just generic explanations, but I feel this is some important knowledge that the Lord wants his people to be aware of in these days.

Let's start by reviewing these nutrition facts.

Proteins-- Are one of the major food groups. They contain essential nutrients which promote growth, strength, energy, weight loss, and more. Common sources of protein include poultry, eggs, beef, milk, cheese, and protein bars or shakes.

Carbohydrates – Are another major food group. There are two kinds of carbohydrates, simple carbohydrates, which are known as sugars… and complex carbohydrates which are known as starches. Sugar is found in foods such as chocolate, honey, candy, cakes, etc. Starches are found in foods like pasta, potatoes, bread, rice etc.

(Basically ANYTHING white or yellow is a carbohydrate)

Now let's look at these hormones in our body.

Insulin - Is the hormone secreted by the pancreas that works to regulate the carbohydrate (sugar) metabolism in the body.

Glucagon - Is a hormone secreted by the pancreas as well. When blood sugar levels are LOWER, glucagon enables the body to tap into its fat stores to USE the stored fat as energy, thus producing weight loss.

So let's sum this up:

<u>Summary</u> - Carbohydrates consumption causes insulin to be released. Insulin takes the excess sugar out of your blood stream to prevent the toxic effects of elevated blood sugar and puts the excess sugar into fat cells to be stored.

However, lower carbohydrate consumption causes glucagon to be released, which promotes the mobilization of (or "burning" of) previously stored fat.

Alrighty. . .

Now I'm not an expert, I'm just explaining this in layman's terms the best I can. But the bottom line is this.

For the most part, your body only uses one of two things for "fuel" or energy. Either the sugar or carbohydrates that you feed it, or stored fat!

So if you're trying to get rid of the stored fat on your body then, that's the fuel source you want to use! Amen?

Let me rephrase that for clarity like this.

Sugar and carbohydrates trigger an insulin release which INCREASES STORED FAT. But a low sugar and carbohydrate supply, triggers glucagon release, which BURNS STORED FAT!

So a LOW sugar and carbohydrate supply is what we need to

focus on to make the physiological fat burning process that God set up in our body work!

And look, I am not a hard-core fanatic about this -- I promise you I am not! There are some folks who decrease their carbohydrate intake so low that to me it's almost seems dangerous. So please don't think I am advocating some extreme way of eating here.

But, let's think!

If *this* is the way God made our body to work. . . and if lower carbohydrate consumption causes glucagon to be released which promotes the burning of stored fat...then, wouldn't it just make sense that you should TRY to eat in a way that works "hand in hand" with that fat burning anointing you are praying for?

You're praying it forth in the Spirit realm...and because you are, you need to be open to doing the things in the *natural* realm that are in harmony with what you're praying forth!

You see to me, it's just wisdom, that as you pray for the things we talked about, that you will then want to listen to the Lord and get your instructions on how to work *with* his power and *not against it!*

**CHURCH, THE HOLY SPIRIT WANTS US TO KNOW THE NATURAL LAWS THAT GOD HAS PRE-SET INTO**

## OUR BODIES!

He does not want us to be ignorant of how our body works, but instead He wants us informed about these principles! Why? Because that enables Him to better lead us in the things that will cause us to lose weight.

And the truth is, that the natural pre-set principle that God has placed within our body is that, carbohydrates IN EXCESS (sugar, bread, rice, potatoes, pasta) are just not good for us!

And when it comes to weight loss, from a purely physiological standpoint, too much of these are going to stop the weight loss process right in its tracks!

So what's the alternative to that?

Well, you want to try your best to avoid carbohydrates and instead, focus more on lean proteins and green or non-starchy vegetables as much as you possibly can.

And let me just throw this in here for lack of a better place.

The "keto" diet is a big thing these days, but with keto they suggest a lot of high fat meat and, that you stay under 20 carbs a day. Now to me, that much fat is just not good for us. And also to me, I feel that low of a carbohydrate intake is just not a realistic change that you can continue for the rest of your life.

But again, you're going to have to get with the Lord and do

what *you* feel led to do. So I'm not telling you to do ANYTHING specific.

I just mentioned keto because as you study this and maybe get online to see what "diet plans" are out there, you're going to come across that term a lot, so you need to be familiar with it.

I mention it too because I do want you to check out the recipes!

There are tons of keto recipes that you can find online (check Pinterest!) that will show you ways you can cook casseroles and everything else under the sun in a way that makes them "low carb"!

And I say that, because once you start thinking along these lines, you'll find there's tons of ways you can cut your carbohydrate intake AND increase your protein intake!

And while yes, you're be eating under the direction of the Lord…at the same time, it's just wisdom to be mindful. Mindful to the truth that restricting your carbohydrate intake and increasing your intake of healthy protein IS the physiologically "weight loss friendly" way of life! Amen?

Now. . .because protein does the opposite of what carbs do, and it is so important, let me add something else I highly suggest.

Protein powder!

Friend let me suggest you make Protein powder a part of your life! You see, I am a huge fan of protein powder because I believe it has been a crucial part of my weight loss journey.

Now I just buy the large tubs of protein from Walmart or Target that cost around $18 and these last me for quite a while. So you don't have to spend huge amounts of money on this. The one I use, has 30 grams of protein with only 3 grams of carbohydrates per scoop! But let me remind you to check the label. You don't want to buy one that has a lot of carbohydrates per scoop. Those are the ones used by body builders to GAIN weight.

But with a low carb per scoop protein powder, you can give yourself huge amounts of protein in a tasty little drink and that protein is going to keep your feeling full. And, it's going to help to get that glycogen activated to help burn that stored fat.

So let me tell you what I do, but again, you do what you feel led to do, ok?

The kind I use, can easily be mixed with a spoon into liquid but you can add all sorts of stuff and use the blender if you want. And for the liquid you can use water, coffee, milk.... (you don't want to use anything with a lot of sugar though) but really any liquid will suffice. However here's what I usually do. (Now I know I'm going to get in trouble from some folks here but just hear me out).

You see I drink, water, water, water by itself all day. And, if I'm not drinking water, I drink unsweet tea with stevia, which is an all-natural zero calorie sugar substitute. But. . . for my protein drink, I use a diet drink. ( I'm sure some of you just cringed!) Now if you don't drink diet drinks, that's fine. I respect you. But the Holy Spirit has not told me not to use a diet drink for my protein, and when He does, I'll stop,

So for my protein, and only for my protein, what I do, is pour some Coke Zero or Diet Dr. Pepper into a big, tall cup and put a scoop of protein powder in it and mix it up!

Now I prefer chocolate. But vanilla flavored protein powder is tasty too, and if you add it into Coke Zero, it tastes just like a coke float only with no sugar and a ton of protein benefits.

You could also use Diet Root Beer and it will taste like a root beer float. Or, you could use Diet Big Red and get the strawberry flavored protein for a really tasty drink as well. There are all kinds of combinations you can mix up according to your taste preference so if you feel led to do this, just make up the protein powder + zero sugar drink combination that you like!

But I telling you, telling you, telling you, that you need to make protein powdered drinks and shakes a part of your life!

Why? Because it's the fastest and easiest way to ingest a large amount of healthy protein. One scoop of protein has approximately the amount of protein as a medium sized steak or a large chicken breast or piece of fish!

And you can mix it up, drink it down, and run out the door and be full for hours! While at the same time giving your body the protein it needs to repair and build your cells and cause your body to burn fat!

Now I mentioned in an earlier session that the Holy Spirit may put it on your heart to substitute some meals with a protein shake because that's what He did for me. I had a lot of weight to lose when He directed me to start adding Protein drinks to my eating habits. And He would often put it on my heart to have a protein drink in place of one of my meals.

And truthfully, if you really want a quick start for rapid weight loss, pray about maybe going 7 or 10 days, or maybe even 21 days having a protein shake for breakfast, a nice Holy Spirit led lunch and then another protein shake for your dinner. Friend, I promise you this is not that hard to do!

In fact, did you know that when folks get the lap band surgery, they have to go on a liquid diet for a pretty long period of time before their surgery (two weeks I think!) where they can eat NO SOLID FOOD and ingest ONLY liquids! (Fun fact: For most of us, if we just did *that,* we would lose a good portion of the weight we wanted to lose! Yipes!)

But I'm not suggesting that. . . I'm really not! I'm just trying to make a point. And it is, that these folks have to have a "liquid only" diet for a long period of time to get this surgery and they all survive! So guess what?

You are not going to starve to death if the Lord prompts you for a period of time to replace your dinner with a protein shake!

So just pray about it.

Because once you get a mixture of the brand and flavor you like and how you like to fix it, I bet the Holy Spirit will prompt you to have that often, as He leads you down the path of supernatural weight loss in your life!

And you know, I was made aware of this years ago, reading an article about a Hollywood actress who had to lose a lot of weight quick for a movie.

And in the article, it mentioned that they made her have 3 protein shakes a day. And then she just ate healthy in between those shakes for her meals. And when they were interviewing her, she had lost like 30 pounds in 2 months or something, and she said that after having 3 protein shakes a day she was so full she barely ate anything else, even though she could have whatever she wanted.

So *that* peaked my interest, I studied it out, and have been a believer in protein shakes, ever since!

So think protein, protein, protein! Because in the world of

weight loss, I like to say that "protein should be your best friend!" In fact, let me give you a little "game" to play concerning your eating.

When you go out to eat, or begin to prepare a meal at home, pray and ask the Holy Spirit, "how can I get the MOST PROTEIN from this meal"?

You see you need to think with natural wisdom. . . *and* pray before you order/prepare. . . and see if the Lord isn't prompting you to make some changes.

( I just saw a quote on Pinterest that said, "If you eat what you've always eaten, you'll weigh what you've always weighed!" ha-ha)

But that's true! You see, if you're used to (just by "default") ordering something like, chicken alfredo or even a hamburger and French fries, often times there is a better, more weight loss friendly way.

Let's me explain and let's think this through.

With those 2 meals as our example, what would be the protein to carbohydrate ratio?

With chicken alfredo, you've got maybe a small chicken breast and / chunks of chicken, so that's like, oh say roughly, 30% of your meal. . . and then you've got this HUGE portion of pasta (which is going to break down to sugar and turn into stored fat) and **THAT** makes up about the other 70% of your meal. And knowing what you now know about the effect of carbohydrates VS protein affecting your weight situation, a 70% carb to 30% protein ratio, is not really a **WISE** weight loss friendly choice.

And think of a hamburger and French fries. Now if you're like me, you grew up on hamburgers and French fries but again, let's think this through. At most fast-food places, you've got a skinny little piece of meat (the least amount they can possibly get by with) and this mini patty is your protein (which is maybe 20% of your meal). Then you've got a great big bun (which is bread, so it's carbohydrates) and French fries which are more carbs! So what's your carb to protein ratio there? **NOT** a weight loss friendly one for sure!

And what's worse, is if you wash it down with a sugary drink. Which amounts to the sugar form of carbohydrates going practically right into your blood stream. . . which is going to cause insulin to be released to open up your fat cells to push all the extra calories right in!

And look, I get it. I eat fast food a lot! But there are ways to do fast food **SMARTER** than the average person does. One who doesn't have the knowledge of how the body works **OR** the direction of the Holy Spirit!

For me personally, usually I feel led by the Spirit to either get a bunch of chicken strips or nuggets (if I'm rushed) or a grilled chicken sandwich, which is usually a big serving of nice lean protein that often comes on a wheat bun (which is lower in carbohydrates than a white bun). Then, I will have just **A FEW** fries. Just enough to enjoy that yummy greasy, salty taste with my meal! 😊

In fact, let me give you a public service announcement here that I never knew growing up. Did you know you don't **HAVE TO** eat **ALL** of your fries? I grew up in the era in which my parents would make us finish everything put in front of us because there were "starving children in China" who didn't have food. Did you ever hear that growing up? I still don't know how me overeating and getting fat helped the children in China, but according to my mother it did!

But one day I found out that if I don't eat all of the fries that they serve me, the world doesn't stop turning. So while I love them as much as anyone else, I try my best to eat the fewest amount of them that I can. And for me, the same goes with other high carb side dishes. Rice, Mac and cheese, mashed potatoes, etc. Sure, you want to enjoy life and not be a weirdo, but no one but you and the Holy Spirit will notice if you just take a few bites.

Now if we are at home and let's say having burgers, I may either have it open faced, with only one side of the bun, or sometimes, I just have two hamburger patties with cheese on a plate and maybe add a nice salad or even pork rinds (no carbs) for my "crunch"!

I mean if you're in the privacy of your own home, no one cares if you're eating kind of weird so you can eat how you want, right?

So here's the bottom line.

**IF YOU WANT TO LOSE WEIGHT YOU ARE GOING TO HAVE TO MAKE SOME CHANGES!** And one of the most important change you can make is to decrease your carbohydrate consumption as much as you can!

But you don't have to be legalistic about it and make a big scene all the time. You want to be able to go with the flow, especially if you're eating out with others and just be subtle about your changes. Because in reality from here on out, you'll be keeping your personal eating strategy your little secret that stays between just you and the Lord. Amen?

## SUGAR, SUGAR

Friend if, in the world of weight loss, protein should be your "best friend" . . . then do you want to know what, in the world of weight loss, should be your worst enemy? SUGAR!

Let's discuss.

Carbohydrates (bread, rice, pasta, etc.) remember are not conducive to weight loss because they *break down* to sugar. So what I want you to realize today is that sugar. . . just straight up sugar. . . is worse!

Do you mind if I go on a rant for just a second?

Friend, I believe with all my heart that sugar is one of the enemy's main weapons that he uses against us!

I mean think about it. We don't smoke, we don't drink, we don't do drugs, but we eat sugar like there's no tomorrow and we wonder why we have to be asking for healing all the time!

Now some may call me a fanatic, but I am telling you, sugar is deadlier than we think!

I am convinced that too much sugar is terrible for our bodies! Look with me at this verse:

## Proverbs 25:16 Easy-to-Read Version

Honey is good, but don't eat too much of it, or you will be sick.

It's right there friend! Understand please that in Bible times, they did not have refined sugar like we have today, so honey was their source of "sugar". But think about what this tells us!

Now yes, sugar is delicious, sure it is! But so is that worm that a fisherman puts on that hook, to catch that big fish! Amen? (Poor analogy I know!) The worm on the end of a hook, is a TRAP…because the fisherman wants to catch and kill that fish, right? Well, look at this:

## Proverbs 23:1-3 Amplified Bible

When you sit down to dine with a ruler,

Consider carefully what is [set] before you;

For you will put a knife to your throat

If you are a man of great appetite.

Do not desire his delicacies,

For it is deceptive food [offered to you with questionable

motives]

Church, I want you to catch that phrase "deceptive" food!

This implies, there IS "deceptive food" out there, that is, as it reads, "offered to you with questionable motives"!

Hmm. . . who do you think would offer something to you with questionable motives?

The enemy, that's who! The same one who wants you overweight, out of shape, out of breath and opening doors with your choices to diseases that can destroy your health!

Now again, I hate to sound like a loony tune here or some super spiritual eating fanatic. Because I promise you I'm not! But someone has to shake the Body of Christ and cause us to WAKE UP in this area!

We are eating ourselves into premature graves by just mindlessly continuing to make bad food choices without any wisdom or direction from the Holy Spirit. And what the Body of Christ needs to realize is, that the over consumption of sugar is one of the WORSE choices we can make!

Now to be fair, I will say that yes, I believe the Lord *allows* us to enjoy some sugar for special occasions. Birthdays, Holidays, celebrations, etc. sure, have fun! I mean there were times of "feasting" in the Bible to celebrate special events and Jewish Holy days, so yes, I'm not saying you can *never* have sugar. I'm just saying we have to be aware of our sugar intake and use our brain!

The verse that we read from Proverbs 25:16 says, that if you eat TOO MUCH of it…. you will be SICK!

So let's think about that.

You know, experts say that Cancer *feeds on sugar.* Do you want to feed any possible cancer cells in your body? NO, of course you don't!

Also, aside from cancer, we also know that sugar *greatly* contributes to diabetes, right? I heard a man preaching recently and he mentioned that when he was 17 years old, the Lord spoke to his heart to not eat sugar. He's in his 50's now and he said that every member of his immediate family has diabetes, except him!

I thought that was AMAZING!

Understand please that I love cake and cookies and pie and such as much as anyone else. But my thoughts are that as Christians, we need to be aware of the negative effects of sugar. And that it's just a wise idea to "save" our sugar consumption for special occasions only… IF, the Lord gives us the ok to eat it even then!

Why am I so adamant about this?

Because I believe the enemy KNOWS how bad the over

consumption of sugar is for us and that's why he tempts us with it so much!

And if you've heard me teach this before, you know that I like to draw attention to the truth about Halloween.

Now we know that Halloween is basically the devil's big day, right? And we know that everything about halloween is about evil and death, correct? Well. . . what's the *other* main thing that Halloween is "about"?

What it is, that the kids dress up to get and thus, overindulge in, on this day?

SUGAR!    STRAIGHT UP SUGAR, right?

Church, please see the connection here!

Halloween isn't about protein, or vegetables or healthy fruit, is it?

It's about candy! Which is pure sugar that practically goes straight into our bloodstreams!

And how many of you know that high blood sugar, kept high for long periods of time can cause death? (That's why diabetes is so serious... right?)

But again I'll try to be fair here and say, a piece of candy or two for a special treat, every once in a while, is *not* going to hurt you.

But I've seen kids, Christian kids, with giant bags full of candy at Halloween (the devil's high holy day) just sit and eat and eat and eat until they make themselves sick! And I hate to tell you this, but I've seen Christian adults do this too! (As a Youth Pastor I helped put on A LOT of "Fall Festivals"!)

But church, WE need to be smarter than that!

We've got to start to recognize these eating related tricks of the enemy! HE HATES US! And he wants us sick and overweight and miserable so that we're not as effective as we could be for the Kingdom of God!

And to bring it back into this context let me say, that for effective weight loss and weight loss maintenance, for the most part, sugar should NOT be a part of your everyday life!

Church, too much sugar causes chemical changes in your body, that clouds your thinking, makes you extremely tired and even affects your appearance.

In fact, let me suggest that you do an experiment. Now you don't really have to do this. It's NOT part of this program! But if you don't believe what I'm telling you, I'm just saying that if you DID do this, you would see that what I am saying is true.

On one day eat, almost ALL lean protein and green vegetables or salads with lots of water. Maybe have eggs or a protein shake for breakfast, a nice big salad for lunch and a grilled chicken breast or two with some green beans or broccoli or something like that.

Then, after you eat THAT way . . . the next morning, look closely in the mirror at your appearance and take note at how you feel during the day.

You're going to look lean and vibrant. You're going to feel light and energetic. And you'll also feel stronger and more emotionally ready to conquer whatever comes to you that day!

Ok now, on another day...eat NOTHING BUT bread, potatoes and sugar- filled junk food. Just fill yourself up with sugar and carbs and wash it all down with sugar filled drinks.

Maybe have a couple of donuts for breakfast and have like a big plate of cheese covered French fries for lunch. Maybe throw in a big bag of M and M's for an afternoon snack and have a big plate of spaghetti and plenty of garlic bread for dinner with a nice big piece of pie for dessert.

Now, then THAT next morning. . . after you have gorged on carbohydrates and sugar, look in the mirror and take note again at your appearance. And also take careful note of HOW YOU FEEL that next day. I promise you, you're not going to like it!

Sugar and too many carbohydrates, puff you up and make you bloated and doughy looking! Your face will look swollen and dull, your rings will be tight, and your clothes will feel uncomfortable. Plus, the extreme insulin spike that you caused will make you to feel completely exhausted! You'll be sluggish and grumpy and moody for pretty much that whole next day!

## THAT'S THE POWER OF YOUR FOOD CHOICES FRIENDS!

And while that sounds crazy, it's a biological, chemical and physiological truth! This is how our bodies work! This is the way God designed our endocrine system! And this is what we've been doing to ourselves and what the devil doesn't want us to figure out!

But we've got to stop!

Friend, you are a free will being. And you can CHOOSE to eat anything you want! But I believe it's time for Body of Christ to start making better choices. And I'm on a one-woman campaign to see that this information gets out!

Sooooo. . . having gotten that off my chest, let's turn a corner here and discuss something else.

Let me make another suggestion now, just because I think it's a wise one.

Of course you pray about this and if the Lord doesn't give you a green light OR it just won't work for you that's fine. However, I just want to throw this out there because it's something I believe in, and it's this. Intermittent Fasting.

Intermittent fasting is an eating pattern that cycles between periods of fasting and eating. It doesn't specify which foods you should eat but rather WHEN you should eat them.

And here's the deal. You can Google this and people are doing this like crazy for weight loss.

But let me share my take on it. FASTING IS OURS CHURCH! We as Christians are the ones called to fast, because the Bible tells us to do so! Look with me at this:

### Matthew 6:16-18 The Passion Translation

"When you fast, don't look like those who pretend to be spiritual. They want everyone to know they're fasting, so they appear in public looking miserable, gloomy, and disheveled. Believe me, they've already received their reward in full. [17-18] When you fast, don't let it be obvious, but instead, wash your face and groom yourself and realize that your Father in the secret place is the one who is watching all that you do in secret and will continue to reward you openly."

There are two things I want you to notice here. First of all in this passage, we see Jesus, himself saying to his disciples, "WHEN you fast". Which implies that we're *supposed* to be fasting! Amen?

Notice, Jesus doesn't say, "*if* you fast". No. He says, "*when* you fast" meaning, the rest of His point is referring to when you do it!

Now the next thing I want us to glean is, that Jesus says, 'don't let it be obvious…wash your face, groom yourself…" In other words, don't make a big show of it, right?

But look at how this ends. He says, "the Father. . . who is watching…will "reward you openly"! Wow!

That's reason enough to fast right there, huh? Praise the Lord!

So my question is, *why* don't we do it? Well let me give you my take on that.

I feel it's because once again, the enemy has tricked us. He has connected a negative connotation to the word "fast" and misled us into thinking that fasting basically implies not eating anything for 40 days!

So because we subconsciously equate it to practically being in a concentration camp, we mentally shut down at even the suggestion. Why? Because it scares the majority of the Body of Christ to even think about! Amen?

But look. What if fasting could be in small increments? Like just not eating anything after say, 7 o'clock at night, until the next morning?

I mean that's doable, huh?

You're going to be asleep most of that time, so you probably won't starve to death between 7 pm and the time you go to bed, right?

Ok, then, hold that thought and let's take this back to the context of weight loss.

You see, "intermittent fasting" is all of the sudden becoming a big "weight loss" thing.

You can do an internet search of that term and get tons of stories and suggestions about it from worldly people and worldly sources. And "they" are all into it not for spiritual purposes, but as one of the new, "cool", weight loss fads!

And to me that is remarkably interesting. The fact that 'they" have discovered how good this is for one's body AND how it helps to keep ones weight issues in check.

Because what some of these internet weight loss guru's do, is simply take a certain time at night and decide not to eat anything after that time, until a certain time the next day.

They may say, "I do intermittent fasting from 6PM to 10AM the next morning".

Or, "I do an intermittent fast from 8PM to 8AM the next day."

And I'm really cracking up that they think they discovered

some new thing, but yet, I'm really saddened by the fact, that it wasn't the Body of Christ who made this known to the world!

But anyway. . . let me just make two points about intermittent fasting here because I DO want you to pray about possibly incorporating some form of this into your life.

Number one. It's just WISDOM to not eat late at night.

In my first book, "Supernatural Fitness", I suggested to not eat after 7PM, because 7 prophetically means "completion" in the Bible and I truly just feel like our eating should be "complete" by 7PM every day.

Why?

Because God made our metabolism to just naturally begin to "shut down" at night to prepare our bodies for sleep. Therefore, anything we eat late at night is pretty much not going to be used or burned up as fuel, so it goes straight into the old storage unit as fat!

However, as with everything else I've suggested, you have to do what the Lord tells YOU to do. But to me it's just not a wise thing to eat late!

Now for those that absolutely HAVE TO eat late for various reasons on certain nights (dinner meetings, family get togethers etc.) let me suggest a strategy that will help "minimize the damage" just a bit.

If you must eat late for social purposes, just don't have any carbs! No bread, no tortilla chips ( we are obsessed with TexMex food here in Texas!) no baked potatoes or French fries, no pasta etc., and certainly no sugar or desserts!

The wisest thing (and the most weight loss friendly thing) you can do if you *have* to eat late is to only have "lean and green" type foods. Healthy lean protein (fish, grilled chicken, etc.), non-starchy vegetables (broccoli, salad, green beans, etc.) and a non-sugary drink!

You can do this folks! Just pray, ask the Holy Spirit what to order and tell the waitress! It's really just that easy! And I promise you, no one will even notice *or care!* However, you and the Lord will have your little "secret"... and you will know that you are working with Him to eat in a way that won't cause you to gain weight! Amen?

Having interjected that, let's now go back to discussing intermittent fasting,

The second point I want to make about this is, that while "the world" is doing it to lose weight (and it does indeed help in that endeavor) I want to suggest that you do this in some form, because of the added spiritual value that it brings to your life!

Church, we know this!

The Word of God tells us that when the disciples couldn't cast a demon out of a man, that Jesus said, "this kind can only go out by prayer and fasting". (Matthew 17:21) So the truth is, that fasting increases our spiritual power!

Do you have a prayer need that you've been praying for, for years AND do you need to lose some weight?

Well then maybe. . . you need to begin to incorporate some form of fasting into your life! So pray about this and see if the Lord puts it on your heart to maybe, not eat anything after 6pm, or after 7, or 8. . . or whatever!

And if your schedule varies, it may need to be different for different days, but here's the deal. If you feel like the Lord is prompting you to stop eating after a certain time, then that is a fast!

So as you claim it as that and attach your faith to it, not only will it facilitate your weight loss but also, you can use this act of fasting to bombard heaven with those prayer needs in which you desperately need to see breakthrough!

So let's say, He puts it on your heart to stop eating at 7pm and you're used to having a late-night snack.

Well, if the Lord has led you to do this, then after 7 when you would normally reach for food, just say no!

Say out loud, "I claim this as a fast and pray forth. . . (my child's deliverance or the breakthrough in my finances or for my husband's job situation, etc., etc., etc.)!

Fasting is Biblical friends!

And the funny thing is that the world just figured out that it helps you lose weight! And it does. . . but WE know it can be used in this other way as well, right?

You see, I feel it is like a "two-sided coin". Its power is both Spiritual AND natural! It actually GIVES YOU an increased level of spiritual power and, less food intake just naturally helps you to weigh less! Which makes it a "win-win" for the Christian trying to lose weight! Amen?

And truthfully, it's not hard at all to make yourself stop eating after a certain Spirit led time in the evening. It's really not!

In fact, it will be supernaturally easy because you'll be empowered by that Anointing of Self-control you are praying forth AND it will supercharge your prayer life as a result!

Now let me interject this here.

None of this is meant to be legalistic in any way! If you go out to eat with your family every Saturday night God knows that. He may prompt you to stop eating at a certain time during the weekdays and do something different on the weekends. This is ALL to be completely between you and the Lord, so just pray and see if He leads you to do this in any way and then go with that! Amen?

Ok, now let's wrap this chapter up by talking about supplements.

Now I don't know if water is considered a supplement, per se, but for lack of a better place to discuss it, I'm going to include it here.

Church. . . YOU KNOW you're supposed to be drinking a lot of water, don't you? But how many of us as Believers really are?

And I don't mean to put condemnation on you but again let the Holy Spirit convict you here if need be!

Because on this program, I am exhorting you to begin drinking lots and lots of good, pure filtered water. Why? Because drinking lots of water is part of your battle strategy against the work of the enemy as you begin your journey of "warfaring the weight"!

And I won't go into a long-detailed thesis on this subject, but I do want to remind you of a few things.

Drinking water helps boost your metabolism which means you burn more fat!

Also it cleanses your body because it flushes out toxins you take in daily through the air and preservatives in your food and such.

In addition to this, it also acts as an appetite suppressant!

You know they say . . . now I don't know who "they" are. . . but they say it, so it must be so. . . but "they" say that sometimes we aren't really hungry, we are actually thirsty. And if we just drank more water, we wouldn't feel the need to always want something to eat! So there's that! 😊

And friend know too, that because there is so much salt in our food these days, drinking lots of water is a good way to combat that issue as well. Water will help flush that salt from your cells which will cause you to lose those extra pounds of water weight. And **THAT** will always causes you to feel better! Amen?

Now, here's a little suggestion I like to make when I teach this information.

Buy yourself a water bottle/or big cup that you love!

I like to suggest those 30 ounces Yeti type cups because they keep your water cold and they are so easy to personalize in a cute way that makes it reflect **YOU!**

I have a white one with a big gold crown on it and that's my cup! Everyone in my family knows it and it's fun to have my big old off brand yeti (lol) to take with me every day.

And you may use a good, filtered water source or buy bottles of filtered water, but however you do it, I suggest that you **MAKE YOURSELF** drink **AT LEAST** 3 of these 30-ounce cups of water each and every day!

Now this is just a general recommendation (because 3 is the number of the Trinity so it's easy to remember and aim for) but as with all of this, you do whatever you feel led by the Lord to do.

However. . . . just please, please just do it! As you begin your new weight loss / health journey I strongly urge you to begin to **MAKE YOURSELF** drink sufficient amounts of water every day just like you would make yourself take some form of medicine that you needed!

Why? Because in a sense, that's what it is. It is "medicine" that improves **EVERY PART** of your body in more ways than we even know!

You see, your body is composed of 60% water and if you don't keep your body hydrated it can negatively affect your major organs and really all of your body systems. So I encourage you to make drinking of lots and lots of water part of your new "arsenal", as you warfare against the enemy's scheme to negatively affect your health!

Ok, now. . . I want to mention a few "vitamin" type supplements that you may want to think about incorporating into your new lifestyle. But remember my disclaimer in that previous section.

Please study this out, talk to your doctor, and pray!

Because I am just sharing some of my personal favorites, but what you ingest into *your* body must strictly remain between you, your doctor and the Lord. Ok?

The first thing I suggest you look into taking is a good multi vitamin.

You see, the way our food is processed these days, it is often pretty much vitamin depleted. So a good multi-vitamin provides you with important trace minerals that your body desperately needs.

Plus there are various forms of vitamins that are known as "anti – oxidants" (Google that). And these antioxidants vitamins have been shown to prevent diseases such as cancer and to help combat aging. Which to me, makes it just a wise thing to look into, Amen?

And your basic antioxidants are:

Vitamin C, Vit. E, Selenium and Beta Carotene

Now for weight loss, there are 3 natural supplements that I recommend but only after you study them out and make sure there are NO contra – indications for these with your health!

The first is some form of Green Tea. Green Tea is simply a natural source of caffeine which causes an increase in your metabolism which will help to increase fat burning.

The next one I highly recommend is coconut oil. (I take the capsule form.) Coconut oil is super good for your skin, plus it's a source of what's called, "Medium Chain Fatty acids". These are said to increase your metabolism and the fat burning process also. Too, it's a healthy source of what they call "good fat", which causes you to feel fuller so that you subsequently eat less!

Now, the last one I suggest you look into is called Garcinia Cambogia. It's made from the peel of the Garcinia fruit and it is said to suppress the appetite, decrease the production and retention of fat in your body and supposedly lower cholesterol and triglycerides. That quality alone makes it a great blessing for your overall health.

So study these out, check with your doctor and pray. Then see if the Lord directs you to start supplementing with these OR any other vitamins and herbs which may be beneficial to you personally.

# STRENGTH!

In the previous chapters I had started discussing the next part of the Daily Prayer and how you will ask for the various anointings. And we discussed the Anointing of "weight loss" and then the Anointing of self-control.

Next if you remember, I explained that by following the prayer (there are copies at the end of this book) that we first, receive the various anointings and then, after receiving them, we follow that with a decree, declaring what that anointing will do. So I want to now discuss with you the next anointing and then explain that particular decree.

The next anointing you will ask for is the Anointing of Strength.

And this part of the prayer looks like this:

*I receive your Anointing of Strength today and I decree that I am strong and energetic, and I exercise how you direct me to in Jesus' name!*

Look with me at this.

### Isaiah 40:29 (New English Translation)

He gives strength to those who are tired;

to the ones who lack power, he gives renewed energy.

Isn't that translation awesome?   And guess what? This is true!

Do you remember when we discussed the spirit of tiredness earlier?

Well the truth is that the enemy would love to make us all so tired every day that we just plop on the couch after work and sit there. . . letting our arteries harden and the extra weight settle in until it's time to fall exhausted into bed! Amen?

But church, I want you to know today, that by receiving the Anointing. . . which is, **GOD'S POWER** for strength and supernatural energy... that strength is going to be there!  And I'm telling you're going to be amazed at the new level of activity you begin to incorporate into your life!  Let's look at another verse.

### Colossians 1:29 out of the Amplified Bible

For this I labor [unto weariness], striving with all

the superhuman energy which He so mightily

enkindles and works within me.

Oh my goodness, don't you love that?

The Holy Spirit's power gave Paul "SUPERHUMAN ENERGY"! That's how the Amplified Bible translates it anyway! But doesn't that verse excite you? It should. . . because that's what you will now be tapping into!

Church, Jesus IS "superhuman", and the Anointing of the Holy Spirit is "superhuman"! So having "superhuman energy" CAN BE a part of your life, IF, you just pray it forth!

I need you to know today, that God's strength is real, tangible, spiritual substance! And as believers we can pray it forth as often as we need it, to supercharge our body! Hallelujah!

I can't tell you how many mornings, when I had to wake up extra early, I would lay in bed and say, "I receive your supernatural strength Lord, I receive your supernatural strength. . ."

And then after just a short time, it's like something "dropped" out of Heaven into me. And I would feel a surge of supernatural energy, that enabled me to jump out of bed and start my day!

So please, please grasp the power of what I'm sharing with you here. Our simply praying for and receiving whatever it is that we need from the Lord makes it ours -- and strength is something that most of us need every single day!

Look with me at this:

### Hebrews 11:11 New King James Version

By faith Sarah herself also received strength to conceive seed, and she bore a child when she was past the age, because she judged Him faithful who had promised.

Are you seeing it?  By faith, Sarah RECEIVED STRENGTH!

So if Sarah could "receive strength" from God to conceive a baby at 90. . . then we can *sure* "receive strength" to get off our behinds and exercise!  Amen?

And friends, spiritually we need to understand that our having strength is so important!   Look with me at this:

### Isaiah 63 Living Bible

Who is this who comes from Edom, from the city of Bozrah, with his magnificent garments of crimson? Who is this in royal robes, marching in the greatness of his strength?
"It is I, the Lord, announcing your salvation; I, the Lord, the one who is mighty to save!"

Church, Jesus IS the epitome of strength!   Think about that!  Everything about Him exudes and exuded strength - both now, how He is in Heaven AND what we know about His life and how he lived when He was on the earth!

Yes, Jesus is *the perfect example* of mental strength, emotional strength, AND physical strength. And as disciples of Jesus, *we* are called to emulate Him and walk in the quality of great strength too!

We are called to be mentally strong! We are called to be emotionally strong! And because we are supposed to be taking care of our bodies, God's temple, we are called to be PHYSICALLY STRONG as well!

That's what this whole program is all about! It's not about "looking good"! It's about God's people becoming LEAN, STRONG AND HEALTHY FOR THE GLORY OF GOD!

And since strength is such a cornerstone of this goal, we have to understand that we have the Anointing of strength freely available to us. And we can and will have it, by simply taking the time to pray it forth!

In fact dear reader, truthfully, we have EVERYTHING we need to lose weight available to us right now! It's all in God's omnipotence, through the person of the Holy Spirit. And the incredible thing is, that all we have to do, is use our faith to pull it "out of God" and into our lives!

It's so easy. . . but we just don't do it!

However from this point on, we are going to be purposeful in receiving what we need from God and through our prayer, we'll receive those attributes of power that will cause us to lose weight!

So again, this part of the prayer goes like this:

*I receive your Anointing of Strength today and I decree that I am strong and energetic, and I exercise how you direct me to in Jesus' name!*

Ok…let's talk about the decree part.

You are going to decree here, "I AM strong and energetic…" But let me stop right here and remind you of the power of your words.

Believer, I want to exhort you to stop saying, "I'm tired" all the time! We all do it, some more that others, but let me suggest to you, that your constantly SAYING it, may be part of the reason you are always so tired!

So, from now on, even if you are feeling that way, try, try, try your best NOT to speak it! Instead, when you recognize in your body you are feeling tired, purposely, take that as a cue to RECEIVE THE ANOINTING OF STRENGTH AGAIN. And maybe receive it over and over a few times and then, out loud make the declaration, "I AM STRONG AND ENERGETIC JESUS NAME! Amen? Amen!

Alrighty, having said that, let's look now at what the rest of the decree says. It says,

*I am strong and energetic, and I exercise how you direct me to in Jesus' name!*

Wait, what? We have to exercise? Yes kids, on this program you still need to exercise! 😊

You see of course, God's power COULD burn all the fat off of your body tonight as you sleep if He wanted to, sure. But don't you know that, as with everything in the Kingdom of God, we still have to do OUR part?

For instance, you may pray and ask the Lord to enable you to win souls.... and God wants you to win souls! But you still have to go out PHYSICALLY to the "highways and byways" and share the gospel, right? Well it's the same with supernatural weight loss and exercise - we have to work in harmony with what we are praying forth!

Remember we are called to be good stewards of our bodies. And to do that, in this earth's realm, it takes exercise. However, as with everything else on this program, I suggest you pray and seek the Lord as to what and how much of that exercise He directs you to do. In other words, your approach to exercise is to be the same as your approach to your new eating habits. Whatever He says to you DO IT! Amen?

Pray about this. . .

He may lead you to join a gym or get a personal trainer (an

actual human) to help you work out.

He may lead you to join the YMCA and do water exercises in the pool or take an aerobics class.

He may lead you to buy a treadmill or a stationary bike or start to follow some exercise DVD's or YouTube workouts at home.

I know a lady who lost over 50 pounds doing the old "Sweating to the Oldies" workouts every day in her bedroom. She never left the house but got a great full body workout, right there at home!

Maybe He'll put it on your heart to start jogging or walking at your local school track or just around your neighborhood. I truly don't know what He will lead you to do, but the bottom line is this.

The Holy Spirit knows what you can do, what you will like, and what will work best for you in **THIS SEASON** of your life! Remember He's a genius. . . a weight loss genius! So keep asking Him and I promise you He'll show you a way you can keep your heart and lungs strong and also work your muscles, as He leads you down the path to greater health.

Because friend. . . let's think about this.

The truth is that we have "morphed" into a society of **SITTERS.**

So many of us sit all day at work and then come home and sit in front of the TV or the computer all night. And, with the little spurts of free time we get during the day, we usually sit and entertain ourselves with our phones, right?

So the bottom line is, that we are *way too sedentary*! And can you see how that could be a trick of the enemy too?

Remember how the enemy works. He puts suggestions in our minds and hopes that we'll agree with those suggestions and act upon them, right? Well, let's dissect satan's strategy.

If we come home from work and THINK (and say) "I'm so tired. . . I just don't feel like getting off the couch. . ." then guess what? We won't get off the couch, will we? So I exhort you today to begin to be consciously aware of these thoughts and actively work against them every day.

Meaning. . . with the anointing that will now upon you, I plead with you to stop agreeing with the enemy's sedentary, lazy, slothful suggestions, and *instead,* start to purposely think about how you will now begin to *move your body as much and as often as you can!*

With your free time, instead of vegging out in front of the computer...think, "what can I do to be active?" And then, clean the house, mop the floor, walk the dog, work in the yard – whatever form of activity that pops into your mind! Anything is better than nothing church, so just move, move, move as much as is possible every day!

Maybe begin the habit of walking around the block every evening after dinner or purposely park further away at the mall. You know, when I weighed almost 100 pounds more than I do now, I can't tell you how many times I went around and around and around the Walmart parking lot. . . looking for a close parking spot, so I didn't have to walk very far! Ugh!

But now, I park way down towards the end of the parking lot and see it as exercise. Wow – what a difference the strategies of the Holy Spirit can make!

Anyway. . . we really just need to increase the movement of our bodies in every way we can, because the truth is, we sit *way too much!* And I don't know all the ways you can increase your physical activity (because the possibilities are endless) but I assure you, if you will just put a conscious effort towards doing your part, God will meet your efforts with His blessing and supernatural power!

But back to exercise. . .

Let's talk about the specifics of exercise just a bit.

Exercise for the most part, can be divided into two categories. The first is what they call "Cardio" or aerobic exercise.

And the generic "Google" definition from the Harvard Medical School website is this:

Aerobic exercise is the type of exercise which speeds up your heart rate and breathing. It is important for many body functions and gives your heart and lungs a workout and increases endurance.

Aerobic exercise also helps relax blood vessel walls, lower blood pressure, burn body fat, lower blood sugar levels, reduce inflammation, boost mood, and raise "good" HDL cholesterol. Combined with eating less, it can lower "bad" LDL cholesterol levels, too. Over the long term, aerobic exercise reduces your risk of heart disease, stroke, type 2 diabetes, breast and colon cancer, depression, and falls. One should aim for 5, 30-minute sessions per week of moderate-intensity activity. Try brisk walking, swimming, jogging, cycling, dancing, or classes like step aerobics.

Ok. . . now the other basic type of exercise is called resistance or weight training exercise. Let's see what the folks at the Harvard Medical School say about that. The article reads:

As we age, we lose muscle mass. Strength training builds it back. Regular strength training will help you feel more confident and capable of daily tasks like carrying groceries, gardening, and lifting heavier objects around the house. Strength training will also help you stand up from a chair, get up off the floor, and go upstairs,.

Strengthening your muscles not only makes you stronger, but also stimulates bone growth, lowers blood sugar, assists with weight control, improves balance and posture, and reduces stress and pain in the lower back and joints.

A strength training program should be done two to three times a week and will likely include body weight exercises like squats, push-ups, lunges, and exercises involving resistance from a weight, a band, or a weight machine.

Church, here's the deal.  Exercise has SO MANY BENEFITS!

And in addition to those we just mentioned, exercise increases the release of endorphins, which are the feel-good hormones in our bodies, that serve to displace depression and stress!

Also, exercise increases the blood flow to your brain, which improves your memory and gives your mind more clarity.

And in addition to all of that, exercise will ultimately increase your self-confidence!  Because it makes you feel stronger, leaner, and just better about yourself overall!  So with all that said, let me just say exercise is one of the best things you can do to improve your overall health – so can you see why the enemy will do ANYTHING he can, to keep you from it?

Selah... 😉

Let's pivot just a bit now and let me share with you some thoughts about the best TIME to exercise. Now, all exercise is good, of course.

But. . . if you remember in a previous chapter, I told you that for the most part, the body only uses one of two things for fuel or energy.

It either uses carbohydrates you have eaten _or_ stored fat.

Therefore, in a perfect world, the _ideal_ time to exercise is when your carbohydrate supply is depleted. When you've already used all the carbohydrates you have eaten as fuel. In other words when you are hungry. Because if there's no sugar or carbs to burn for energy in the old storehouse, your body _has_ to tap into those fat stores for energy -- and thus, burn fat!

Which is our goal, right? So.... when would that time be?

Well, ideally, the best time would be first thing in the morning on an empty stomach!

You see, after you have slept all night, any carbohydrates you ate the day before, have pretty much all been used up by your body for energy and the "storehouse", (my descriptive word, not a real thing! Ha-ha!) then is on "empty", so to speak.

Random fact: That's why they call that first meal of the day "break-fast". Because you are "breaking" the "fast" . . . the time that you were asleep and *not eating* during those sleeping hours.

Also, interesting side point. What are the majority of breakfast foods composed of? Carbohydrates! Right? Cereal, toast, bagels, orange juice (which is super high in sugar) pancakes, waffles, breakfast bars, etc., etc., etc. . . . So think. What does the average American do as soon as they wake up? Replenish their carbohydrate stores, for the body to use for energy! However, in doing so, they don't give their body the chance to burn fat!

But. . . if you can get up and jump on that treadmill or go to an early morning exercise class or take a bike ride around the neighborhood etc., if, you can do some form of cardio exercise on an empty stomach, **YOUR BODY WILL BE FORCED TO TAP INTO YOUR FAT STORES AND START BURNING THAT EXTRA FAT ON YOUR BODY FOR FUEL!**

Then... if you will eat only protein for your breakfast (a protein shake, eggs, eggbeaters if you're watching your cholesterol, maybe with some type of breakfast sausage, etc.) you won't be replenishing that carb supply just yet -- so by combining the exercise on an empty stomach **WITH** a protein only first meal, your body will be burning fat for the first couple of hours of the day!

And then when lunch rolls around, you can have some nice, yummy carbohydrates! (Because you do need carbs! ) So personally, I highly suggest you make lunch your biggest carbohydrate rich meal of the day.

However, back to my point. All exercise is great, yes!

But your choice of **WHEN** to eat carbohydrates in relationship to **WHEN** you exercise, can and will greatly increase the effectiveness of your weight loss when it comes to burning fat.

So again, you do what the Lord leads you to do, but my personal suggestion is early morning exercise and a protein only breakfast meal.

Now, I know a lot of folks hit the ground running each morning, and I get that. . . but just pray about this and see if there is any way you can work this in.

I know of a pastor who says he gets up and jumps on his treadmill, for the first 30 minutes of his morning, before he starts anything else that day.

Also, I know a lady who is a teacher, who has to start getting ready at 6AM for school. She told me she has an exercise bike in her garage and that she gets up at 5:25, goes straight into her garage, cycles for 30 minutes, and then jumps in the shower right at 6 to start getting herself ready for school.

So there ARE ways you can do this, but *if*. . . it's still just impossible for you, I understand that too! So let me give you my second suggestion as to another great time to exercise. If you can't get up early, try this.

Let's say you eat lunch every day at 12 and you work until 5 PM. Well, by 5, any carbs you consumed at lunch are pretty much used up. That's why you're dragging when you walk out the door!

But IF. . . instead of going straight home and eating dinner. . . you could work your exercise in at THIS time. . . (as long as possible AFTER lunch but BEFORE DINNER) you're still pretty much "on empty" as far as carbs go.

So if you can go to an exercise class, or stop by the gym, or change your clothes at work and go to the track or the mall to walk BEFORE you eat dinner, then the same principle will kick in! It's been like 4-5 hours since you ate, so your body is going to have to find that fuel somewhere. And if you're a bit hungry, it's going to be using that stored fat to get the fuel (the energy) to do whatever it is you are making your body do.

And then ideally after that, if you would eat basically a high protein and non-starchy vegetables (no corn, no carrots, no potatoes, no rice, etc.) meal for dinner, you won't be restoring your carbohydrate supply and your body will continue to burn fat throughout the night!

Remember, it's you AGAINST the extra weight on your body

and this is the way the Lord made our bodies to work. If you exercise on a carbohydrate empty stomach, physiologically, it makes your body burn that extra fat! Amen?

Let me remind you that this is warfare church! Spiritual warfare yes, but because you're in a natural body it's warfare in the natural realm too!

And as in any warfare, it's imperative that you know your enemy! And that you know what empowers and dis-empowers that enemy so you can plug into that knowledge to make your warfare effectively work!

You see a big part of the problem is, that the majority of Body of Christ doesn't exercise. And I know that Paul said in 1 Timothy 4:8, that "bodily exercise profits little" but that's not an excuse, not to do it. Because what Paul is implying there is, that natural exercise, IN AND OF IT'S SELF, doesn't have eternal value. But, we have to realize that the good stewardship of our bodies, through the USE of exercise, DOES! In fact, look with me at this passage:

### 1 Corinthians 9:24-27 New Living Translation

Don't you realize that in a race everyone runs, but only one person gets the prize? So run to win! All athletes are disciplined in their training. They do it to win a prize that will fade away, but we do it for an eternal prize. So I run with purpose in every step. I am not just shadowboxing. I discipline my body like an athlete, training it to do what it should. Otherwise, I fear that after preaching to others I myself might be disqualified.

Intercessors, prayer warriors, ministers and mature believers, are we really grasping what this says? Listen closely to those words. "I DISCIPLINE MY BODY like an athlete, training it to do what it SHOULD. Otherwise, I fear that after preaching to others I myself might be DISQUALIFIED."

Disqualified? WHAT?!?

Guys, could Paul be telling us something here that we all too often overlook? That disciplining and training our body to do what it SHOULD do, is supposed to be a part of our Christian life?

Will we be held accountable to God one day for how well we walked this out in our life? I don't know. . .

But look, again, the Lord is not asking us to be body builders and beauty queens. He just wants us to TRY! To try to do whatever it is that we *can do*, on whatever level we may *be on*, to make exercise an unnegotiable part of our life.

So just pray about this and let the Lord lead you. Amen? Amen!

Now let's turn a quick corner here as we finish up this chapter. Because now, I want to quickly go over the last anointing that you will pray forth each day to assist you in achieving supernatural weight loss in your life. And it is, the Anointing of "fullness"! And here's how that part of the prayer goes.

*I receive your Anointing of Fullness today and I decree that I stay supernaturally satisfied in my appetite in Jesus' name!*

Let's discuss.

Now this one too, is not something that's just obviously mentioned in the Word of God. But like I've said, I've sought the Lord on this subject for a lot of years and I believe He's shown me some truths that we can tap into here.

Look with me at this:

### 1 Kings 19:7-9 International Standard Version

Later, the angel of the LORD came a second time, grabbed him, and said "Get up! Eat! The journey ahead is too difficult for you!" [8] So Elijah got up, ate and drank, and survived on that one meal for 40 days and nights as he set out on his journey to Horeb, God's mountain.

Now… it doesn't say so exactly here, but I am surmising from this that Elijah *probably* didn't get ravenously hungry for that 40 days. Because evidently the Angel made that one meal sustain him *supernaturally* for all that time!

And this may seem like a bit of stretch to you, but in my mind he may have been given what I would call an "anointing of fullness". And that's what we will be praying forth every day too, by following the daily prayer.

And really the proper scientific word is "satiety", which means, "the quality or state of being fed to capacity and/or feeling full". But to me, not many of us use that word, so I just say "fullness". Because I know the Lord can do this for us *if* we simply ask!

You see, this is the opposite anointing that we need to combat that "excess hunger and food cravings" spirit that we talked about earlier. And I'm am telling you with my hand up to the Lord that this works!

And what prompted me to study this out was because years ago, when I was developing this prayer strategy in my head, the Lord kept having me hear people say, "I'm always hungry".

Like it almost got comical. Everywhere I went, during conversations I would have with people at church, at football games, etc., it seemed like during this time, in the course of talking, I would hear people say things like, "well, I can't help it, I'm just always hungry". Or, "I don't know what's wrong with me it seems like "I'm always hungry". Or, "I just can't diet, because I'm always hungry. . ."

And I agreed with them every time because it seemed like I was "always hungry" too!

However, after a while I got to thinking.

Wait...this isn't a 3rd world country... we are middle class American people with plenty of access to food. WHY do we THINK, SAY and FEEL like we are "always hungry"?

Hmmm...? So being the "always searching for clues, weight loss detective" that I am, this made me suspicious!

So that's when I started to pray forth what I felt was the opposite of that, which is fullness. And as soon as I did, I started seeing this anointing work powerfully in my own life!

So the bottom line here is, that if the Lord can cause Elijah to go 40 days without starving to death after one meal. . . then He can cause us to stay satisfied in our appetites so that we are not constantly thinking we *need* something else to eat!

Friend, by binding that spirit of "excess hunger" that we discussed earlier and praying forth the "anointing of fullness", your appetite is going to be supernaturally diminished in Jesus' mighty name!

Look with me at these verses.

## Psalm 63:5 New Living Translation

You satisfy me more than the richest of foods.

## Psalm 145:16 New Living Translation

When you open your hand, you satisfy the hunger and thirst of every living thing.

Church notice what these verses are showing us here.

## GOD HAS THE POWER TO SATISFY YOUR APPETITE SUPERNATURALLY!

And I'm telling you, I'm telling you, I'm telling you, when you pray this forth every day, IT'S THERE!

You'll find yourself, missing meals because you just forgot to eat!

You'll find yourself not wanting those "habit snacks" you used to have to have because you just don't think about them anymore!

It's really the coolest thing, I promise you! But because you are spiritual leaders, let me close this chapter with this.

Being around "ministry people" for years, I've noticed an interesting phenomenon. Many, many ministers fast before their service so that the anointing will be on them really strong.

And look, I've been to hundreds of special conferences and services and I've never heard one minister say that they were HUNGRY while the service was going on!

You see they are preaching or teaching and then often times praying for folks for extended periods after that, and during the time that they are *under the anointing*, eating and food, is the last thing on their mind!

However, when that anointing lifts and the service is over, understandably many ministers then go directly to the nearest restaurant to eat. Why? Because once the anointing has lifted, they are now feeling hunger again. And the first thing they want to do is satisfy that NOW discernable urge.

So here's what that tells me. I get it. I have fasted before I would preach or teach and know that it is a necessary spiritual discipline. However, what I want you to understand is the underlying hidden truth that we see here at work.

The Anointing quenches hunger! Under a heavy anointing one is just *not* hungry! So let's catch this powerful truth and comprehend how we can apply it to our lives.

If the anointing is able to quench or suppress hunger during ministry, then *why can't it suppress hunger at any other time?*

I'M TELLING YOU IT CAN!

The power of supernatural "fullness" in your appetite is *in* the omnipotence of God church! And we can "pull on" that God quality if we just know about it... and pray if forth!

And that's what we will be doing when we receive the Anointing of fullness each day!  And then we will follow that by decreeing that our appetites stay "supernaturally satisfied", which will not only cause us to eat less at each meal but will also greatly decrease all those in between meal snacks as well!

**Praise the Lord!**

## COMMUNION

Good news! We are coming into the home stretch here and you're almost ready to begin "warfaring the weight"! Yay! But first, let's review your Daily Power Prayer and then I'll explain what you do next.

Every morning you'll pray something like this:

*In the name of Jesus, I take authority over every demonic spirit affecting my body, my weight and my health and I render these spirits POWERLESS to operate in my life in Jesus' name!*

*Spirit of Heaviness, Spirit of Overeating, Spirit of Tiredness and Spirit of Excess Hunger and Food Cravings, I bind you, I break your power, I command you to leave me now in Jesus' name!*

*Holy Spirit I ask you today to be my Personal Trainer.*

*Lead, guide and direct me in my eating and exercise habits and empower me to lose this extra weight and become supernaturally healthy, in Jesus' name!*

*I bless my body today Lord, and call it lean, strong and healthy...*

*but I curse the extra weight on my body and command it to "be removed and cast into the sea"!*

*I receive your Anointing for Weight Loss today Lord, and I decree that I am lean in Jesus' name!*

*I receive your Anointing of Self-Control today and I decree that I eat only what and how much you direct me to eat in Jesus' name!*

*I receive your Anointing of Strength today and I decree that I am strong and energetic, and I exercise how you direct me to in Jesus' name!*

*I receive your Anointing of Fullness today and I decree that I stay supernaturally satisfied in my appetite in Jesus' name!*

Now that took like, maybe a minute or so to read, right? So I promise you, you can do this. . . because if you do, it will be one of the most spiritually profitable minutes of your day!

But after you pray that, you're going to do something next that is going to put the final nail in the enemy's coffin so to speak, concerning your weight issues.

You see every morning, after you pray the daily prayer we just went over, you are going to "seal the deal" by taking communion.

Now before you give up on me here, and think, "I don't have time to do that every day" just hear me out! Because I promise you that what you're about to begin to do, has more supernatural power than many of us have realized. And IF...you will simply follow through with this, the Lord will **SUPERNATUALLY TRANSFORM** both your body and your life!

However, before we start, I need you to brace yourself because you are going to need to have your "big girl/ boy pants" on here, to hear my explanation. It's not an easy comparison to put out there, but it's the truth none the less. Let me explain.

There is a mighty man of God that I listen to often on YouTube. He preaches in some wonderful churches and has an incredible testimony in that, he was radically saved out of a lifestyle of a satanic cult. In his various teachings, he mentions periodically some of the things that the "other side" does to obtain Satanic power. And while I won't go into all the detail, let me generically share this truth to make my point.

When the witches / warlocks / satanists want to increase their level of demonic power, they do various "rituals" - most of which involve some sort of sacrifice and the shedding of blood.

Now again, we know that the devil only COPIES real spiritual truth. Nothing he has or does was created by him, he simply perverts and twists the things and truths in the Kingdom of God. But what we can glean from this is that when "they" do these things, true spiritual power is released. Albeit, it's the enemy's power, it's demonic power... but through the ACT OF THEIR RITUALS...supernatural power, is actually and tangibly released!

And I shared that not to glorify this travesty in anyway, but instead to hopefully make you understand this.

When *they* do these types of things, (involving sacrifices and blood) the reality is, that they are mocking the act of taking communion and the spiritual power of the flesh and blood of Jesus Christ. Their "counterfeit" actions releases real "counterfeit" power.

Which tells *us*. . . that they know a truth that you and I need to know and make use of, purposely, in our Christian life.

The act of communion, when done properly releases power. It releases real, supernatural, tangible GODLY power. And believe it or not, that power can be targeted, to achieve overcoming victory in the weight problem area of your life!

Now to me, it's a shame that I had to discern the true power of communion by finding out the ways and actions of those who hate my Lord and Savior Jesus Christ.

You see by realizing the power their "mock" communion released, it made me see and understand the TRUE Godly power that our Holy Communion will release.

Because the reality is, that there is power in the act of taking communion beyond what we can imagine! I believe it is a greatly misunderstood ordinance that we think is just a sweet little act that we do, to "remember" Jesus. But church, it is much, much more! Look with me at this.

### John 6:51-56 New King James Version

I am the living bread which came down from heaven. If anyone eats of this bread, he will live forever; and the bread that I shall give is My flesh, which I shall give for the life of the world."

[52] The Jews therefore quarreled among themselves, saying, "How can this Man give us His flesh to eat?"

[53] Then Jesus said to them, "Most assuredly, I say to you, unless you eat the flesh of the Son of Man and drink His blood, you have no life in you. [54] Whoever eats My flesh and drinks My blood has eternal life. [55] For My flesh is food indeed, and My blood is drink indeed. [56] He who eats My flesh and drinks My blood abides in Me, and I in him.

Now, if you think about it, that's some pretty shocking

sounding stuff Jesus was saying there. And the funny, but not funny thing is, that if you continue to read that passage, in verse 66 it says;

From that time many of his disciples went back and walked no more with him.

How sad is that? Because He said something that sounded so "off the wall" many of His disciples left Him! They were like, "yeah. . . He was good when He was healing folks, but then He said we are supposed to eat His body and drink His blood, so...umm. . . I'm outta here!"

Now I admit this does sound a bit gruesome, but if it was out of the mouth of Jesus then it contains spiritual truth. And that truth IS… that His Body and His Blood contain power and He wants us to "eat" and "drink" of it. And while that sounds wrong on the surface, actually, he was letting us in on a little secret here, that would not be fully understood until after His death.

And that truth is, that we can "re-release" the power of His Body and His Blood into our lives through the prophetic act of taking communion! And Church, this is something we need to be made aware of so that we can plug into it every day for the rest of our lives.

Communion releases power!  Real, tangible, supernatural, transformational power!

Communion expresses the spiritual truth of Jesus' death, resurrection and victory over every work of the enemy!  And it prophetically "reactivates" the finished work of Jesus on the cross!

And the reason we will do it on *this* program is to release that supernatural power into our weight issues, our bodies and our health!

You see, as we say here in Texas, "this ain't my first rodeo"! I've studied and taught on the subject of health and weight loss for many years.  And when I first got this revelation about communion as it pertained to my weight problem, the Lord explained it to me like this.

He showed me that the original sin came into Adam and Eve through the act of eating. . .

And that the enemy has put us in bondage to our weight, through the act of eating. . .

And that, **WE CAN TURN THE TABLES ON THE ENEMY AND SET US FREE IN THIS AREA THROUGH THE ACT OF EATING!**  The "eating" of the elements of communion... *if* we take of its power and apply it to this area of our life!

So friend here's the truth.

As Believers, if we take communion each day following the prayer we are praying to help us overcome our weight issues, we can add to the power of that prayer *by imparting the victory of Jesus' finished work on the cross into this particular aspect of our lives!*

And when we do this, it will in time, transform our bodies supernaturally. Because it's power will be activated to make us lean, strong and healthy for the Glory of God!

Isn't that exciting?

Know this today.

When you partake of communion, a spiritual impartation takes place. An impartation of His triumph over the work of the enemy and an impartation of His physical well-being into YOUR body and life!

You see, communion gives you an impartation of all that Jesus is and all that Jesus accomplished, being prayed directly into our weight loss efforts, our bodies and our health!

I mean, is there *anything* more powerful than the finished work of Jesus? No! There's not! And that's what you can be "taking in" each day as a follow up to your daily prayer.

Think of it this way.

It's comparable (although weakly, I'm sorry!) to downloading a program onto your computer or downloading an **APP** on your phone.

Every time you partake of communion, you are "downloading" spiritually, Jesus' physical wellbeing into your overweight, unhealthy body. And in time, the spiritual substance of Jesus' leanness, strength and health will work supernaturally, to bring about some wonderful changes in this area of your life! Praise the Lord!

Now... let's discuss some of the specifics.

There are many ways you can do this because truthfully the particular elements that you use are really not that important.

You may want to buy some disposable communion packs online or, you may just use a pinch off of a cracker and some juice.

I used to always use a piece of a Frito (lol because it's just what we always had handy) but now I buy a box of those little round soup crackers and simply use one of those.

Also, I know people who use grape juice, cranberry juice, soda, water and even coffee for the liquid. And while I know these may sound a bit "sacrilegious" . . . truthfully, what you use does not really matter at all. It's the ACT that matters, *not* what you are ingesting. So please, just find something that's easy for you to have available every day.

Another suggestion I want to make is that you say the prayer and take your communion in the morning before you really start your day. And I know mornings are usually rushed and that we often hit the ground running and race out the door trying not to be late for work. But, IF you can just make time...I promise you it will be worth it! Because you want the power of the act of taking communion, to be working within every aspect of your day.

Ok, so with all that said, let's take a look at the communion aspect of your daily prayer.

It goes like this:

### Communion

*Jesus, I take of this bread, as a supernatural impartation of YOUR body. I decree that this impartation is going into my body and is supernaturally transforming my body to be lean, strong and healthy like yours.*

*I receive now, your body into mine. (Take of the bread)*

*Jesus, I take of this juice as a supernatural impartation of YOUR blood. I decree that this impartation is going into my body also, and it's breaking the power of the enemy off of my body and imparting into me, leanness, strength and Divine health.*

*I receive now, your blood. (Take of the juice)*

As you see, again, this is pretty much self-explanatory.

By following along ( but feel free to change the wording however you feel led to) what you will be doing is, taking the "bread" (in whatever form you have available) and the "juice" (in whatever form you have available) and going through the act of taking communion each day, targeting the power of this holy action towards your body, your weight loss battle and your health.

Now, I am not going to write a detailed explanation about the taking of communion in general, because hopefully as a Believer, you are already familiar with this. If not, there are plenty of good books out there written by great spiritual minds for you to study. And if you aren't knowledgeable about this subject, I do suggest that you study it out on your own.

But to sum this up, for our purposes here, I just want to say, this works!

I wish there were words to adequately express the supernatural power of God that is released when you take communion in this way, but there aren't. It is such an incredibly precious and exciting thing, that all I can say is just to try it yourself to see the results.

Also I don't want anyone to think I am taking the act of communion lightly here because I am not. I suggest you examine your heart each morning before you partake and also, repent and forgive anyone you may have aught against as well. The fear of the Lord and a sense of His holiness is *always* the proper way to enter into this act and just because you will be taking it every day, that doesn't change.

But. . . with that said, once you begin your communion process each day you need to know and believe the enormity of what will now be taking place.

Your taking of the "body of Christ" with true heart felt belief in the power of what Jesus bled and died for you to have, actually creates a supernatural transformation process that is unexplainable to the natural man.

Our God is a supernatural God friends! The resurrected body of Jesus Christ and His shed Blood have more power than anything on this earth! And this act, of "remembering" His sacrifice, actually releases the spiritual truth and substance of who and what Jesus IS and what He DID! And it's time for us as Believers in Jesus Christ to know, understand and tap into this truth.

The power of taking communion can transform ANY area of your life! Now on this program I suggest we target it towards our health and our weight battle, but please know that if you are dealing with other problems and/or attacks of the enemy you can apply it to those areas too!

Church, when you take by faith, the "Body of Christ" into your body and your life, you are spiritually receiving an invisible impartation of Jesus' body into yours!

And when you take by faith, the "Blood of Christ" you are doing the same. But let me say this about that.

When I was in the 9th grade, I had to do a research paper on the Circulatory System. (Eye roll!) But the bottom-line conclusion that I never forgot was, that as blood runs through our circulatory system it does two things. It removes "toxins" and brings forth healing or "new life".

So it is also with the Blood of Jesus. Jesus' Blood is so powerful and it's power is actually two-fold. It removes the "toxins" of the work of the enemy. . . and it brings forth healing or the "new life" of Jesus' victorious resurrection.

That's how we will use Jesus' Blood represented through communion on this plan.

As the Communion part of the prayer states, you will receive the transformational power of these two elements of communion, intentionally, knowingly and purposefully. And by doing that consistently, you're going to experience not only supernatural weight loss but an entire supernatural TRANSFORMATION of your body and your life! Amen? Amen! Our Lord is so, so good!

Okedokee. . . stay with me for just a bit longer because we are almost done! There is now one more thing I need to explain to you, that I suggest you do as part of this program. And it's incredibly powerful too, so hang on to your hat!

On your Daily Prayer Sheet, at the bottom, you'll see it says "Impartation" and it reads like this:

*Impartation (Lay hands on yourself 3 times daily)*

*I impart supernatural weight loss into my body. . .*

*I impart the fire of the Holy Spirit to go forth into my body and burn off the extra weight. . . .*

*I impart the presence of God that melts mountains, to go forth and melt the extra weight off my body . .*

*I impart Weight Loss Glory into my body and into my life, in Jesus' mighty name!*

Let's dissect this first, and then we'll read it again, so you'll more fully understand. Look with me at this verse:

<u>Mark 16:18 New American Standard Bible</u>
. . . if they drink any deadly poison, it will not hurt them; they will lay hands on the sick, and they will recover."

And out of The Message Translation it reads like this:

## Mark 16:18 The Message

. . .. they will lay hands on the sick and make them well."

Church, how many of us know this truth?

Do we not *know* that the Lord has instructed us to "lay hands on the sick" and pray for them?

Sure we know that! And we *do* that, right?

If someone came into our church service and said, "I'm not feeling well, will you pray for me?" What would we do? We would place our hand on them and pray, correct? Because that's how we roll! That's just what we do! Well, church, my question to you is this. WHY DON'T WE DO THIS TO OURSELVES? Well... for now on, we will!

You see the last part of your Daily Prayer serves as a simple reminder for you to lay hands on yourself, 3 times a day, and **IMPART INTO YOURSELF GOD'S POWER FOR SUPERNATURAL WEIGHT LOSS!**

Now we've discussed "supernatural weight loss" previously but let me remind you of this truth.

There are meetings and services that Believers go to with certain ministers who move in signs, wonders and miracles, and some of them very often have miracles of instant, or supernatural weight loss occur, right there while the people are sitting in their seats! Look this up on YouTube. You can see proof of this with your very own eyes!

So because this happens then let's think. If this is something the Holy Spirit does, then why would we think He wouldn't do it for us?

Especially if we have the faith for it and we purposely, use our faith, to impart it into our bodies every day. So I exhort you to do this! And I personally suggest 3 times a day simply because this is something I do in the morning before I even get out of bed, sometime during the day (just whenever I think about it) and then at night after I go to bed before I go to sleep.

And what you'll do, is simply lay hands on yourself, like Mark 16:18 say, to "recover" (lol) from your weight loss issues, and "make yourself well" in this area so to speak!

And look. . . I know that verse is actually referring to sick people. But how many of us are "sick" of being overweight? ☺


Well guess what? Through the finished work of Jesus Christ, you now have power in your hands! And it can be used for *every* purpose... even this one! So let's use it church! Amen?

Therefore, 3 times a day... lay hands on yourself. And let me show you the verses we'll be pulling on to impart this truth. Look with me at this:

## Isaiah 10:16-18 New King James Version

Therefore the Lord, the Lord of hosts,

Will send leanness among his fat ones. . .

Now remember we looked at this verse earlier and I showed you that word "leanness" there in the Hebrew was the word "razown" and it means to "make thin", right?

Ok, so to read it again it says: (Verse 16)

Therefore the Lord, the Lord of hosts,

Will send leanness among his fat ones;

And under his **GLORY**

He will kindle a burning

Like the burning of a fire.

Let's stop here and talk about this.

On this program, we are going to impart into ourselves, what I call "WEIGHT LOSS GLORY"! And we do that for many reasons. You see, the Glory is God's presence, His power and His personality as it manifest in the natural realm here on the earth. Church, the Glory is all that God is. . . and frankly church, it's *everything* that we could ever need!

And in THIS context, we need, WEIGHT LOSS! Amen?
So we are going to call this aspect of God's Glory, "weight loss Glory" in our impartation because as we read on, we see in this passage that that is exactly what is happening "under His Glory"! Let's look at that again and read a bit further; (verses 16-18 Emphasis mine)

> Therefore the Lord, the Lord of hosts,
>
> Will send leanness among his fat ones;
>
> And under his GLORY
>
> He will kindle a burning
>
> Like the burning of a fire.
>
> So the Light of Israel will be for a fire,
>
> And his Holy One for a flame;
>
> It will burn and devour
>
> His thorns and his briers in one day.
>
> [18] And it will consume the glory of his forest and of his fruitful field,
>
> Both soul AND BODY;
>
> And THEY WILL BE AS WHEN A SICK MAN WASTES AWAY.

Now, remember we already discussed this. That wasting away there, ISN'T SICKNESS! God does not put sickness on a person because there is NO sickness in Him to give!

No, this is referring to a decrease in the size and weight of their bodies. That same kind of "wasting away" that happens *when* one is sick. But here, we see another dimension of this passage in that, all of this is happening, "UNDER THE GLORY"!

And it goes on to say, the Holy one will be a "flame", that will burn and consume their body. . . *so that they will be like when a sick man waste away!*

Now don't let this freak you out, just see the overall truth here.

Church *this* is what we can impart into the extra weight on our bodies! And it's **NOT** death or sickness or disease. It's the fire of the Holy Spirit's power, that we see here, working to make their bodies become thin ("waste away")! It's that Razown leanness friend! It's supernatural weight loss! The Lord is using His Glory like a fire, to release His supernatural weight loss through!

So. . . . what I need you to fully understand today is that YOU can use the power of the laying on of hands to impart this manifestation of God into yourself! We know our hands can be conduits of power, and now that you realize "supernatural weight loss" is a "thing", you can use those hands to facilitate this power for supernatural results!

Do you remember in the movie "The Wizard of Oz", when Glenda said to Dorothy, "you've had the power all along"?

Well that's us, church!

I am telling you with all the conviction I can muster, that as a born -again Believer, you CAN BE lean, strong and healthy by just tapping into the power of God! You've just got to put the principles that affect your health and your weight loss efforts to work!

Let me show you now another verse we'll use. Look with me at this:

### Psalm 97:5 New King James Version

The mountains melt like wax at the presence of the LORD,
At the presence of the Lord of the whole earth.

Ok, fun fact. One touch of the God's presence could turn Mount Everest into a pancake!

He is incredibly merciful to us, because the truth is that God is SO powerful, that if he just thought it, the whole earth would explode into a million pieces if that's what He so desired.

Now He won't do that, because He loves us, but He could...because that's how much power He has!

So look. If you can grasp how much power the Lord really has...and if you can grasp how that power can be released through the laying on of hands. . . then you can easily and effectively put that power to work "melting off" the extra weight on your body that is not God's perfect will for you! Amen?

Well again, that's what you'll be reminded to do daily on your Daily Prayer. Let's look at it again, now that we've gone over the verses that we are plugging into:

You'll say:

*I impart supernatural weight loss into my body. . .*

(Now, remember, this happens in some meetings, so it's not some "out there" impossible thing, right?)

And then you'll say:

*I impart the fire of the Holy Spirit to go forth into my body and burn off the extra weight. . . . . .*

Remember we saw in Isaiah 10, that "the light of Israel will be a FIRE and the HOLY ONE a FLAME" that will "BURN", right?

And also remember Hebrews 12:29 says, that our God is a "consuming fire" so it's not even that much of a stretch to impart this into yourself, because what you will be saying is truth straight from the Word of God!

But then, you'll say;

*I impart the presence of God that melts mountains, to go forth and MELT the extra weight off my body. . .*

Psalm 97:5, the mountains melt like wax at the presence of the Lord, right? And then you'll say:

*I impart Weight Loss GLORY into my body and into my life, in Jesus' mighty name!*

Church, we truly *are* coming into the time of God's Glory manifesting on the earth! And God's people, losing the weight they need to lose so that they are lean, strong and healthy for His Glory is something that the Glory CAN and WANTS to do!

Ok then, guess what?

It's about to start in your life RIGHT NOW in Jesus' mighty name!

Praise the Lord!

## REVIEW

To conclude this teaching I want to tie this this together and put a big bow on it so to speak. So let's start by simply reiterating what you've already (hopefully) learned.

You see on this program you have learned how to "Warfare the Weight". Which is, the extra weight on your body that ideally should not be there. And you do that by every day, praying a targeted prayer *and* taking some spiritually targeted actions, that will cause the Supernatural power of God to be specifically released into your weight issues and into the overall health aspect of your life!

Now this prayer and those actions are outlined word for word for you on your Daily Prayer sheet. And again, there are several copies for you to tear out and have handy at the end of the book, but just for fun, let's take a look at it here. The entire prayer goes like this:

*In the name of Jesus, I take authority over every demonic spirit affecting my body, my weight and my health and I render these spirits POWERLESS to operate in my life in Jesus' name!*

*Spirit of Heaviness, Spirit of Overeating, Spirit of Tiredness and Spirit of Excess Hunger and Food Cravings, I bind you, I break your power, I command you to leave me now in Jesus' name!*

*Holy Spirit I ask you today to be my Personal Trainer.*

*Lead, guide and direct me in my eating and exercise habits and empower me to lose this extra weight and become supernaturally healthy, in Jesus' name!*

*I bless my body today Lord, and call it lean, strong and healthy… but I curse the extra weight on my body and command it to "be removed and cast into the sea"!*

*I receive your Anointing for Weight Loss today Lord, and I decree that I am lean in Jesus' name!*

*I receive your Anointing of Self-Control today and I decree that I eat only what and how much you direct me to eat in Jesus' name!*

*I receive your Anointing of Strength today and I decree that I am strong and energetic, and I exercise how you direct me to in Jesus' name!*

*I receive your Anointing of Fullness today and I decree that I stay supernaturally satisfied in my appetite in Jesus' name!*

## Communion

*Jesus, I take of this bread, as a supernatural impartation of YOUR body. I decree that this impartation is going into my body and is supernaturally transforming my body to be lean, strong and healthy like yours.*

*I receive now, your body into mine. (Take of the bread)*

*Jesus, I take of this juice as a supernatural impartation of YOUR blood. I decree that this impartation is going into my body also, and it's breaking the power of the enemy off of my body and imparting into me, leanness, strength and Divine health.*

*I receive now, your blood. (Take of the juice)*

*Impartation (Lay hands on yourself 3 times daily)*

*I impart supernatural weight loss into my body. . .*

*I impart the fire of the Holy Spirit to go forth into my body and burn off the extra weight. . . . . .*

*I impart the presence of God that melts mountains, to go forth and melt the extra weight off my body. . .*

*I impart Weight Loss Glory into my body and into my life, in Jesus' mighty name!*

Let's review!

First, you will each day, bind the demonic forces that have been (unknowingly by you) influencing you to be too heavy, causing you to overeat, causing you to eat extra food and snacks that you don't really need and causing you to be overly tired and apathetic about exercise.

So once those spirits are bound up. . . you will then, ask the Holy Spirit to lead, guide and direct you in your eating and your exercise choices. Because remember, He is a genius at this, and His directions obeyed will produce supernatural results!

Now next, you will take a second or two, to bless your body and speak forth it being "lean, strong and healthy", but then, you'll curse the extra weight on your body and command it to be removed and cast into the sea!

Next, you will ask for the various aspects of God's anointing to be activated on you that day as you walk this out. These anointings are, the anointing for Weight Loss, Self-control, Strength, and Fullness.

After that, you will take communion each day, applying the power of Communion to your weight issues and receiving by faith, the power of Jesus' finished work in this area.

Then to wrap it up...at some point, 3 times during the day, you will purposely use your faith to lay hands on yourself and impart God's power for weight loss and weight loss Glory into your life!

Now... you will just go on with your day, staying plugged into the Lord, consulting the Holy Spirit as to what and how much to eat AND any exercise that He may direct you to do that day.

You see my sweet friend, this is not a "diet". It's a lifestyle.

A lifestyle of connecting this area of our lives to the power of God and then walking this out by following the Holy Spirit's directions as best you can, making corrections and changes as they are needed, to produce for you a better quality of life!

Remember, that's our goal.

It's not about being a super model or Olympic athlete, it's about coming out of bondage and having peace in this area, while living in a body that you feel good about! Amen?

But before we go any further, let me go back a bit and remind you of some things I mentioned earlier, that I really suggest you do before you actually start.

First of all, remember to get some sort of notebook to write in, so you can keep yourself accountable for a while. Now this won't be a forever thing, because once you live like this for a period of time, you'll just be on auto – pilot with all this. So you won't need a notebook forever. . . but it is a good way to start!

You can put the date and day of the week at the top and just write down what you eat and if and how you exercised that day and if you drank your water and how much.

Also, write down anything the Lord may have spoken to you about all of this (He'll be teaching you all sorts of things as you go along) and write down any revelational truths about yourself and your eating or exercise habits that you discover. (Situations that "trigger" you and make to want to eat, etc.) You see ANY transformation comes with new revelation! So keep these powerful truths journaled so that you can go over it later, pray into it, and train yourself how to do better from here on out!

But before you even do that. . .

Pray and seek the Lord and figure out what you feel the Lord is leading you to do, eating and exercise wise. Because I promise you from the bottom of my heart, that HE HAS A PLAN!

Look with me at this.

### Jeremiah 29:11 New International Version

For I know the plans I have for you," declares the LORD, "plans to prosper you and not to harm you, plans to give you hope and a future.

Church, this verse, applies to *every* area of our lives!

And what I need you to understand today is that God has a plan, that you can seek Him about and follow...that will enable you to lose the weight you need to lose and get healthy!

He really, really does!

But the problem is that we have been walking around thinking we can figure it out for ourselves. . . and then we wonder why we gain and lose and gain and lose and never really come to a place of peace in this area of our lives!

So before you start...SEEK HIM FOR THE PLAN!

Does He want you to follow some "already out there" meal plan or strategy?

Or does He want you to take it "meal by meal" each day?

Does He want you to join a gym or buy a treadmill?

Or does He want you to get your family involved and start a walking program every day?

Does He want you to fast after a certain time in the evening until a certain time each morning?

Or does He want you to eat like normal on the weekdays and fast in some form on the other days?

I don't have a clue what YOUR plan is. . . but I assure you, all the details are IN the plan! And the Lord has the perfect plan/ "strategy" that will be doable, affordable and supernaturally effective just for you!

Have you heard that saying, "Plan your work and work your plan"?

Well your perfect plan is in the mind and heart of God, and you get access to it, by simply seeking Him for it and praying it forth! Amen? Amen!

Ok. Now once you get your "plan" . . .once you get an idea of what you feel like the Lord is directing you to do, then carrying out that plan, becomes what I like to call your "routine".

Let me explain. Look with me at this verse from two different versions.

## Proverbs 29:18 Expanded Bible

Where there is no word from God people are uncontrolled...

## Proverbs 29:18 New Living Translation

When people do not accept divine guidance, they run wild.

Friends WITHOUT some type of plan from God being made into a routine we follow through on, "we run wild"! We are "uncontrolled"!

You see, if we don't place upon ourselves some distinct "boundaries" in these areas, we give the enemy a huge open door in the spirit realm that allows him to come in!

If we don't have this area of our life under some sort of restraint. . . if we don't have any type of prayed forth system or structured "routine" . . . that LACK OF REPETITIVE DISCIPLINE, gives the enemy a way to easily influence this area of our lives.

Lack of a "routine" enables him to just come in and cause you to gain more and more weight and get unhealthier and unhealthier, day after day after day.

Without some sort of pre-determined disciplines. . . a plan. . . your "routine" . . . it's like we have no borders. And the enemy then sees us as easy prey that he can manipulate to steal, kill and destroy our health.

By seeking the Lord and deciding, something like "ok, I'm going to eat thus and thus way every day, and I'm going to exercise by doing this and this on these days of the week" . . . this Spirit led planned routine, makes this area of your life more "structured". Which in a sense, puts "walls around it" so to speak, to help protect your eating and exercise habits from being infiltrated by the enemy who is seeking only to do you harm.

Remember, 1 Peter 5:8 tells us the enemy roams about like a lion, looking for whom he can devour. Yes, he's just looking for those without ANY form of self -discipline in this area so he come in and do his thing!

Church, we've got to come up higher! And we've got to be SMARTER!

The world is kicking our behinds in this area and looking down on us for being in such poor physical shape when we should be lean, strong and healthy to show them the power of our wonderful God!

The Lord just wants us to try friend. *Any* sort of effort in this area is better than none! And *any* effort in this area lessens the enemy's ability to infiltrate our health. So seek the Lord about this and get a plan! And then work your plan and make it your routine!

For instance, let's say you prayed and felt like the Lord led you to follow a low carbohydrate meal plan, to only indulge in sugar on Sunday, and to walk every evening after work, Monday through Friday. Ok, then, THIS is your plan. And as you DO IT, it becomes your "routine".

Therefore, if the enemy tempts you with cake at work on a weekday, you simply say "no thanks", because that's NOT a part of your God-led plan/routine. And if you feel tired after work on Monday, you go and walk anyway, because you (and the Lord) know that this IS a part of your God-led plan/routine.

Now look, again, none of this is meant to be legalistic in any way, but gee whiz church, we have **GOT TO MAKE OURSELVES BECOME MORE DISCIPLINED!**

Because discipline in this part of our life acts as a fortress in the spirit realm to ward off the schemes of the enemy, who wants only to steal your health!

So anyway. . . once you feel like you have an idea of what the Lord is leading you to do...then that's the plan!

And now you can begin to pray your Daily Prayer each day and *walk that plan out as it transforms your life!* Yay Jesus!

You see friends, I believe with all my heart, that God's people should be the healthiest people on the planet!

I believe that we should be exhibiting supernatural Divine health as a sign and a wonder of God's Glory and goodness, and that's one of the reasons why I am so adamant about the use of these ideas.

I feel it's time for us to "reverse the curse" in a lot of areas, and I believe we can do that concerning our bodies.  But to do so, I strongly believe that we have to be consistently praying into this situation and cooperating with the Holy Spirit every day. And that's what this prayer system makes us do!  Amen? Amen!

So....as we begin to wrap this thing up, let me turn a corner here with a closing point. Look with me at this: (Emphasis mine)

<u>Romans 12:2 New King James Version(Emphasis Mine)</u>
And do not be conformed to this world, but BE TRANSFORMED <u>BY</u> the RENEWING OF YOUR MIND, that you may prove what is that good and acceptable and perfect will of God.

Church it's time for us to truly understand the power of our minds.

You see, your thoughts are often formed from spiritual influences that you are not aware of. These (demonic) "influences" want you to take hold of an untrue thought and hold it in your mind as a belief. Why do they do that?

Because your mind is so powerful that if you BELEIVE your thoughts are reality, then your circumstances will tend to shape themselves around that belief.

So to cut to the chase for our purposes here, I'll say this.

If you've had fat "producing" and fat "accepting" beliefs all these years. . . it's time for you to renew your mind!

You see through the finished work of Christ, we are able to transform the *physical* realm, by activating the *spiritual* realm!

Remember, we are actually spirit beings, simply housed in these earthly bodies, so our Spirit man is, what SHOULD be in charge.

But our mind is the device that serves as the "middleman" so to speak!

For instance. . . if your mind believes things such as, "grandma was fat, momma was fat, I'm just fat and I'll always be fat!" . . . well then, BAM!

Guess what?

With all that mental determination, in **THAT** particular belief, then fat you will indeed be!

However. . . if we are wanting to lose weight and feel better about ourselves physically, then the *first* thing we need to do is to **CHANGE OUR THINKING!**

Because the way to break any cycle. . . is to change the beliefs stored in your mind!   In other words, "renew your mind" as it says there in Romans 12:2!

So in our case, what I need you to know today is this:

It doesn't matter if you are 90 years old and you weigh 500 pounds. You can, right here and right now, decide in your mind... that you are well able to be lean, strong and healthy through Christ!

And then, simply start taking the steps and walking out the actions that are in agreement with *that* faith filled belief!

Because by doing so, and believing that this *can* be done, **YOU'LL SEE THE HOLY SPIRIT'S TRANSFORMATIONAL POWER RELEASED FOR *THAT* BELIEF IN YOUR LIFE!**

Church, with the Lord it's really easy. . . but the first step you must take is to simply decide that you believe!

Make that decision and say to yourself something like, "*I have decided to be a health and fitness focused person! I am going to be lean, strong and healthy for the Glory of God and I'm going to use the knowledge and the experience I acquire, to help other people in their weight loss efforts too!"*

Now as we close, let me get deadly serious here for just a second my friend.

I want you to realize that the Lord _needs_ you to do this!

Why?

Because you have an entire sphere of influence that you can help to get healthier! You see, your new knowledge and _your example_ will make them believe that it's possible too!

As spiritual leaders please understand, that as *you* get this area of your life together, you will then want to minister this to others! That's all I've done. Remember the before and after pictures I showed you earlier?

One day I just decided that I didn't want to look or feel the way I did any longer, so I plugged into God's power and didn't stop pressing into Him until I lost all the weight I needed to lose!

So now I'm sharing all this with you. . . and the Lord wants YOU to go and do the same!

And understand this. You don't have to get anyone's permission to become a voice for good health!

And... you don't have to wait and get to a certain size or a certain weight before you start! **START NOW!**

Let the folks in your sphere of influence see you doing it...because that will inspire them to get focused on this area as well!

Which, if you think about it, could be lifesaving for some.

Remember the introduction of this book and how I discussed obesity's direct effect on the various health issues? Church, our being overweight isn't funny. And you as a leader taking a vocal and visual stand for weight loss and better health is actually something that could mean the difference between life and an early death for some. . .

So just decide and believe that you are right now, a health and fitness enthusiast, tapping into the Power of God that *cannot fail* and then watch what happens!

Because as you decide to do this, and then stay plugged into the Holy Spirit, He will see to it that YOUR determination and HIS power brings you to the place of seeing your body and health supernaturally renewed for the Glory of God! Amen? Amen!

Now get busy folks! I'm praying for you! ☺

(PS: You'll find 3 copies of the Warfare the Weight Power Prayer on the following pages. You can keep them in the book to go by or tear them out to keep in your Bible or notebook.)

# Warfare the Weight Power Prayer

In the name of Jesus, I take authority over every demonic spirit affecting my body, my weight and my health and I render these spirits POWERLESS to operate in my life in Jesus' name!

Spirit of Heaviness, Spirit of Overeating, Spirit of Tiredness and Spirit of Excess Hunger and Food Cravings, I bind you, I break your power, I command you to leave me now in Jesus' name!

Holy Spirit I ask you today to be my Personal Trainer.

Lead, guide and direct me in my eating and exercise habits and empower me to lose this extra weight and become supernaturally healthy, in Jesus' name!

I bless my body today Lord, and call it lean, strong and healthy…but I curse the extra weight on my body and command it to "be removed and cast into the sea"!

I receive your Anointing for Weight Loss today Lord, and I decree that I am lean in Jesus' name!

I receive your Anointing of Self-Control today and I decree that I eat only what and how much you direct me to eat in Jesus' name!

I receive your Anointing of Strength today and I decree that I am strong and energetic, and I exercise how you direct me to in Jesus' name!

I receive your Anointing of Fullness today and I decree that I stay supernaturally satisfied in my appetite in Jesus' name!

## Communion

Jesus, I take of this bread, as a supernatural impartation of YOUR body. I decree that this impartation is going into my body and is supernaturally transforming my body to be lean, strong and healthy like yours.

I receive now, your body into mine. (Take of the bread)

Jesus, I take of this juice as a supernatural impartation of YOUR blood. I decree that this impartation is going into my body also, and it's breaking the power of the enemy off of my body and imparting into me, leanness, strength and Divine health.

I receive now, your blood. (Take of the juice)

### Impartation (Lay hands on yourself 3 times daily)

I impart supernatural weight loss into my body. . .

I impart the fire of the Holy Spirit to go forth into my body and burn off the extra weight. . . . . .

I impart the presence of God that melts mountains, to go forth and melt the extra weight off my body. . .

I impart Weight Loss Glory into my body and into my life, in Jesus' mighty name!

# Warfare the Weight Power Prayer

In the name of Jesus, I take authority over every demonic spirit affecting my body, my weight and my health and I render these spirits POWERLESS to operate in my life in Jesus' name!

Spirit of Heaviness, Spirit of Overeating, Spirit of Tiredness and Spirit of Excess Hunger and Food Cravings, I bind you, I break your power, I command you to leave me now in Jesus' name!

Holy Spirit I ask you today to be my Personal Trainer.

Lead, guide and direct me in my eating and exercise habits and empower me to lose this extra weight and become supernaturally healthy, in Jesus' name!

I bless my body today Lord, and call it lean, strong and healthy....but I curse the extra weight on my body and command it to "be removed and cast into the sea"!

I receive your Anointing for Weight Loss today Lord, and I decree that I am lean in Jesus' name!

I receive your Anointing of Self-Control today and I decree that I eat only what and how much you direct me to eat in Jesus' name!

I receive your Anointing of Strength today and I decree that I am strong and energetic, and I exercise how you direct me to in Jesus' name!

I receive your Anointing of Fullness today and I decree that I stay supernaturally satisfied in my appetite in Jesus' name!

## Communion

Jesus, I take of this bread, as a supernatural impartation of YOUR body. I decree that this impartation is going into my body and is supernaturally transforming my body to be lean, strong and healthy like yours.

I receive now, your body into mine. (Take of the bread)

Jesus, I take of this juice as a supernatural impartation of YOUR blood. I decree that this impartation is going into my body also, and it's breaking the power of the enemy off of my body and imparting into me, leanness, strength and Divine health.

I receive now, your blood. (Take of the juice)

## <u>Impartation (Lay hands on yourself 3 times daily)</u>

I impart supernatural weight loss into my body. . .

I impart the fire of the Holy Spirit to go forth into my body and burn off the extra weight. . . . . .

I impart the presence of God that melts mountains, to go forth and melt the extra weight off my body. . .

I impart Weight Loss Glory into my body and into my life, in Jesus' mighty name!

# Warfare the Weight Power Prayer

In the name of Jesus, I take authority over every demonic spirit affecting my body, my weight and my health and I render these spirits POWERLESS to operate in my life in Jesus' name!

Spirit of Heaviness, Spirit of Overeating, Spirit of Tiredness and Spirit of Excess Hunger and Food Cravings, I bind you, I break your power, I command you to leave me now in Jesus' name!

Holy Spirit I ask you today to be my Personal Trainer.

Lead, guide and direct me in my eating and exercise habits and empower me to lose this extra weight and become supernaturally healthy, in Jesus' name!

I bless my body today Lord, and call it lean, strong and healthy.... but I curse the extra weight on my body and command it to "be removed and cast into the sea"!

I receive your Anointing for Weight Loss today Lord, and I decree that I am lean in Jesus' name!

I receive your Anointing of Self-Control today and I decree that I eat only what and how much you direct me to eat in Jesus' name!

I receive your Anointing of Strength today and I decree that I am strong and energetic, and I exercise how you direct me to in Jesus' name!

I receive your Anointing of Fullness today and I decree that I stay supernaturally satisfied in my appetite in Jesus' name!

## Communion

Jesus, I take of this bread, as a supernatural impartation of YOUR body. I decree that this impartation is going into my body and is supernaturally transforming my body to be lean, strong and healthy like yours.

I receive now, your body into mine. (Take of the bread)

Jesus, I take of this juice as a supernatural impartation of YOUR blood. I decree that this impartation is going into my body also, and it's breaking the power of the enemy off of my body and imparting into me, leanness, strength and Divine health.

I receive now, your blood. (Take of the juice)


Impartation (Lay hands on yourself 3 times daily)

I impart supernatural weight loss into my body. . .

I impart the fire of the Holy Spirit to go forth into my body and burn off the extra weight. . . . . .

I impart the presence of God that melts mountains, to go forth and melt the extra weight off my body. . .

I impart Weight Loss Glory into my body and into my life, in Jesus' mighty name!

# ABOUT THE AUTHOR

Pastor, author and Conference Speaker Peggy Lee, has served
the Lord in every church capacity for almost 40 years.
She brings fresh revelation and power to the Body of Christ
through her books, sermons and seminars.
Peggy oversees Majesty Ministries, a ministry dedicated to
empowering Believers to live victorious lives through the truth
of their Royalty in Christ.

CPSIA information can be obtained
at www.ICGtesting.com
Printed in the USA
LVHW081732110221
679064LV00035B/1365